Dear II: For Amaadi
Audrey Adade

To Eddie

Identifiers: ISBN 978-1-304-30791-0 (pbk.) | ISBN 978-1-304-62670-7 (ebook)

Book editor: **Burgeon Publishing**
Book designer: **Audrey Adade**
Cover designer: **Audrey Adade**

Lulu, Inc. www.lulu.com

www.ascwaconsulting.com

TABLE OF CONTENTS

PREFACE

Mental illness does not define who you are. You are more than your illness. I am a writer. I am a social worker. I am a public health professional. Mental illness did not change any of this. I just have something new to write and speak about. As I reflect on the past, I realize I am not my imperfections nor my flaws, nor my negative experiences. In fact, my imperfections and flaws add to my experiences. They have helped me to bless the lives of others. I have accomplished so much in my life. If it had not been for my pitfalls, I would not have been able to do either. I am not a victim. I am a victor. I am powerful beyond measure.

I thank God every day for all of my experiences, both good and bad. The good experiences were fun. The bad experiences built character and strength and made me a living testimony. I want to give back to my community, my country, and to those who I don't know whose stories are just like mine. I want to help them get through the hard moments. I know that not everybody needs to know my story. However, I believe it is very important for everyone to share their stories. We do not go through things for ourselves. We did not suffer because God was punishing us.

Rather, we go through things and suffer to be a blueprint of survival for those with similar struggles. It is selfish to keep our stories to ourselves. We have a responsibility to share our testimonies. There are lives on the brink of ending that can be saved by telling our stories. I am more than what was meant for my demise. There was a plan for my defeat, but I never gave up. The enemy will never have a foothold on me. My backbone is erect and stable as a tree. I have no more tears. I have no more fears. I have no more guilt. I have no more shame.

Jesus is ever-present and near. Never will He leave me to fight on my own. My history has consistently shown. Never will I fall too hard to rise up. Never will the enemy shut this girl up. Faith and hope and promises anew. His will be done. I have already won. I write this through tears because it has been hard. There were many scary moments. Before I knew my purpose, I asked God, *why*. I did not understand why I was being punished. It did not make sense to me. Little did I know, He was by my side throughout it all. When I discovered who He was, I learned that my life had a purpose. I did not suffer in vain. I have touched tens and thousands of lives. I fight for my family. And I fight for those tens and thousands whom I do not know. The enemy lied to me, making me feel like I was all alone.

God sends angels our way to help us. We must use the pain we go through as healing for ourselves and the healing of others. You are more than your illness.

I am Andrea Anastasia Andrews, and I am not ashamed. One year ago, I hit rock bottom and crashed. My psyche hit a concrete wall. My emotions took a turn, and I lost control. I was no longer steering my mind. Fear took over. I was depressed.

Jesus is first in my life. He, my family, and a few loyal friends saw me through the toughest times. He is the One. I opened myself to Him as a teen. When you are young and depressed, you live in a vacuum of doubt and confusion. Life is grim and a chore. Youth means nothing because a heavy burden rests on your shoulders. Darkness replaces the sunshine you once had.

I was hospitalized in a center providing both mental health services and drug rehabilitation. It was there I learned how to trust, love, and express myself. For the first time, I was open. I was among people who had similar stories. Inside that center, there was no stigma in sharing our stories. We trusted each other. I was amazed and surprised at how open people were about their mental health struggles. Despair lifted from me and dissipated. Perfection was no longer a goal; health was now my goal.

Life is not flawless. It is alright to have pitfalls. My pitfall was a breakdown. All the anger I held at the world reversed and bombarded my core. So, I journaled. It was a practice I was used to naturally since middle school. However, at the hospital, it had a different use. It was a coping skill. They told me to journal. Writing was therapeutic. I journaled about the past, present, and future. I created poems like, "Come."

Come now, clarity.
Come now, peace.
Come now, energy.
Come now.

Come now, rationale.
Come now, breath.
Come now, healthy body.
Come now, healthy mind.
Come now, forgiveness.
Come now.

Come now, strength.
Come now, love.
Please stay.

I wanted love. Love meant nurture, freedom, attention, appreciation, happiness, and life. Love was a way out of a vicious mental illness.

Pain: Pain is a hard feeling and a hard place to be. I have known pain for a long time.

Anguish: I often feel exasperated. Anguish comes when you have been through it all or when you feel that way.

Strength: I find strength in God and my family.

Survival: It is a fight to survive in this world. It is a fight when, obstacle after obstacle, you feel beaten. But you are still alive when you pinch yourself.

Faith: Faith holds you together. It puts together all the pieces of the enigma. It sticks like glue to everything and everyone on your spiritual journey, including you. God is always there even when it does not seem like He is.

Tears: Tears flow a lot when you are happy or sad or just flaming hot with anger. Tears can be like therapy without a copay.

Body: Your body represents you.

Life: Life is brief. It should be appreciated. Life should be done right.

Soul: It is your inner being. It is what stays. It is mysterious. Nurture it, and let God in.

Mind: The mind is precious. It is fragile, yet abstract. It is necessary. It is powerful. That is why it hurts to lose it. That is also why it takes so much to do so. This is the beginning of my story.

CHAPTER 1:

EARLY DAYS

It was camp, in 1987. My brother and I were at this lady's house who had way too many children to oversee. We were at the pool. I was feeling annoyed because it was hot and I had to keep an eye out for my brother, according to my Mom. All of a sudden, I see a brown blob bobbing up and down in the water. I said to myself, "What is that?"

To my horror it was my 3-year-old brother drowning in the deep end. I immediately jumped into panic mode. But, my instincts kicked in. I jumped into the water even though I was scared of the deep end. I swam over to my brother and got him out. When we got out, he began to cry. I held him and asked if he was okay. He said yes in between sobs. An adult nearby said something in our direction. My immediate thought was, *why were you not doing anything?* Later, the lady who ran the camp said I took good care of my brother, and I was a hero. I didn't want to hear that. I just wanted my brother to be okay. From that moment on, I knew it was he and I against the world.

Bubble baths with suds reaching my ears, the smell of baked bread, cookies, and cake warmed my heart and comforted my soul.

The sound of clapping to the beat of the rhymes, "Down, down baby, down by the rollercoaster, sweet, sweet baby, I'll never let you go, shimmy, shimmy coco pop, shimmy, shimmy power, shimmy, shimmy coco pop, shimmy, shimmy power, momma, momma sick in bed, she called the doctor, and the doctor said, let's get the rhythm of the ___, let's get the rhythm of the ___," and, "Miss Mary Mack, Mack, Mack, all dressed in black, black, black, with silver buttons, buttons, buttons, all down her back, back, back, she asked her mother, mother, mother for 50 cents, cents, cents to see the elephant, elephant, elephant, jump over the fence, fence, fence." "Slide baby, one, one, one, two, one, two, one, one..." and more. The love between my three best friends and I went unmatched throughout my life.

I remember sitting between Judy's legs as my hair was greased, brushed, and plaited into curvy designs. Though the styles did not last due to not covering my hair at night, they were beautiful. These were the happy sounds, feelings, and sights of my childhood. My childhood was full of care, fun, and beauty.

Life Tastes So Good Life tastes so good.

Breathing, experiencing, being feels right.

Waking up to a new day is a blessing from God.

Life tastes so good.

Counting our blessings every day,

appreciating God's grace, and living,

just living.

Life tastes so good.

Heart beats over and over.

Lungs inhale and exhale.

Eyes see.

Mouth speaks.

Soul feels.
Life tastes so good.

Judy was my Dad's secretary. My Dad, the first black male pediatrician in our hometown, exemplifies hard work, the importance of family, and generosity. He has made many sacrifices to provide stability for his children. He leads our family and loves to bring our extended family together. He is a great historian and educates both young and old on our roots. Over the years, we have seen him work 24/7 to provide emergency care to our family and friends as a physician. He has provided compassionate medical care to people who are uninsured and cannot pay. He taught me the value of being knowledgeable and well-read. I would bring him research and term papers, and he would dictate the history and policy to the point where I almost did not need sources. Lastly, he attempted to teach me how to manage finances and balance a checkbook. We are blessed to have him as a father.

My Dad is quiet, soft, and gentle. He takes everything very hard and to the heart, even when there is a need to express himself. For a long time, I thought my Dad did not love me. It was never the case, but I felt that way since he never expressed his love for me. His way was to buy me material things, save for my education, take us on vacations, and give me pocket money to buy whatever I wanted. His idea of conversation and relationship building was to ask about school and nothing else. I took this to heart. My sensitivity turned into anger in my pre-teens and teens. I isolated myself from my family and became engulfed in the superficial support of my friends. They were my escape from the chaos at home. My Dad does love me. In fact, he loves me more than anyone in this world except my mother. I look like him. We have the same personality. My father would drop anything and do just anything for me. I love his selflessness when it comes to taking care of the family. His whole life is based on us, particularly me and my siblings. He set us up for success. And, he was great for school papers and historical conversations.

"Hey, how's your school project on Marxism coming along, sweetie? Do you need any help?" he said.

"Hi, Dad! Yeah, actually, I could use some help," I said. "I'm trying to understand the core concepts of Marxism and how they apply to society. Can you explain it to me in simpler terms?" My Dad was not simple.

"Of course, I'd be happy to help!" he said. "Marxism is a social, economic, and political theory developed by Karl

Marx. It focuses on the idea that society is divided into two main classes: the bourgeoisie (or the wealthy class who own the means of production) and the proletariat.

"Okay, so it's about the rich and poor, right?" I said.

"Yes, that's one way to look at it," he said. "Marx believed that the bourgeoisie exploited the proletariat by paying them low wages while making profits from their labor. He thought this created inequality in society."

"So, what did Marx argue should be done about this inequality?" I said.

"Marx believed that the working class should rise up to overthrow the bourgeoisie and establish a classless society where wealth and resources are shared equally. He called this a socialist or communist society."

I asked, "How would that work exactly? Would everyone be equal?"

He said, "In a communist society, the means of production would be owned collectively, and resources would be distributed based on each person's needs rather than their ability to pay. The goal is to eliminate social classes and create a society where everyone shares in the benefits and burdens equally."

"That sounds idealistic, but is it practical?" I said.

He added, "Many debates exist about the practical implementation of Marxism. While some argue that it can lead to dictatorships, others believe that it can be applied in a more democratic way. It's essential to consider Marxism's historical context and different interpretations before drawing any conclusions."

"I see," I said. "Thanks for explaining, Dad! This definitely helps me grasp the basics of Marxism. I think I have enough to get started on my project now."

"You're very welcome!" he added. "I'm glad I could assist you. If you have any more questions along the way or need further clarification, don't hesitate to ask. Good luck with your project!"

I used to be happiest in grade school with my three best friends, Yvonne Jones, Nicole Pellini, and Kristen Wells. My grade school years were the happiest times of my life— kindergarten through fourth grade. I was secure in all my relationships, both friends and family, and I had fun exploring the things I enjoyed doing, such as writing, artwork, music, and dance. I enjoyed the school I attended, Saint Cecilia, a coed Catholic school in Stamford, Connecticut. My happiness changed when I hit fifth grade and started at Brooklawn School. I felt the school was cliquey and isolated from the rest of the world. I felt the need to make friends outside of school. There was a strong divide between the students of color and the Caucasian students.

I was a very precocious kid. I remember the days I lived with full abandon, a child full of trust, with a mind full of treasures that dazzled, glittered, and shined. I was free like the wind that greets every crevice in the land. The limitless options ahead, like the endless, rushing waters of the sea, enveloped me. My bright eyes reflected innocent faith in the world around me.

My beloved brother Amaadi is developmentally disabled. I love my brother with all of my heart. Yes, he irritates me, but he is a precious soul. I believe that God brought him into my family's life to test us and make us strong. Everything happens for a reason.

When I look deep into his eyes, I see pain, anguish, frustration, and sadness. He wants so badly to lead a normal life. However, he is trapped within his own mind. Every day that he gets older and bigger, his situation becomes worse. There is no cure. The disease gets worse over time.

Living with a person like my brother takes a large toll on the entire family. We jump at his every move. He gets whatever he wants, whenever he wants. His daily activities are a burden on every other member of the family. We have all reacted to his situation differently. We all have been equally affected by his problems, but in different ways. It is not his fault.

CHAPTER 2

DEPRESSION – MENTAL HEALTH AND CRISIS

Enraged

When I am mad, the world around me is too. The

valleys are barren.

The deserts are extremely hot.

The mountains and the hills are fighting for a place in this bitter world. The world is against me.

I feel self-pity.

For the beauty I once saw is gone.

My lens is clouded where happiness was once seen. My heart is barred from all reasoning.

My spirit is immune to glee. Happiness, please set this captive free.

Depression is a mental health disorder characterized by persistent feelings of sadness, worthlessness, and a lack of interest or pleasure in activities. It is a mood disorder that affects a person's thoughts, feelings, and behavior, leading to a variety of emotional and physical symptoms. These symptoms can interfere with daily functioning and have a negative impact on relationships, work, and overall well-being. Depression can vary in severity, with some individuals experiencing mild symptoms that come and go, while others may experience severe and long-lasting symptoms known as major depressive disorder. It is important to note that depression is a complex condition influenced by a combination of genetic, biological, environmental, and psychological factors, and it often requires professional help and support to manage effectively.

For me, depression is like a vacuum. The illness sucks the being out of you. It feels like there is no end in sight. It engulfs your mind and body like a sponge that only sucks in negative energy. I do not want to go back there again.

Also, depression can be triggered by anxiety and stress. It can also hit you at a low time in your life. For me, it was the last term of my senior year in high school. Everything I did felt like a chore. Sleeping was my only escape from the melancholy that rested in my psyche.

I had a lot of anger towards family and friends over the littlest things. I was an angry and bitter person. It all became bottled up in my body. I felt physically weak. I had no energy to do all the things I normally did. Nor did I have the energy to keep up with friends. Life just felt hard.

I did not trust anyone around me, including my parents, siblings, and friends at school. In hindsight, my depression was mostly based on deep sadness over my relationships with family and friends. I went to private schools all of my life. That had a profound effect on me. I was often the only person of color in my classes or one of a few. My best school experience was in my Catholic elementary school. Back then, I was truly happy with my friends, with my school, and with life in general. Life is different through the eyes of a child. There are fewer external pressures, and the perception of life is more innocent and simple. During my depression, I longed for a return to this state of being.

My worst school experience was the six years after Catholic school when I was a preteen at Brooklawn School. I absolutely hated the environment I was in. Socially, I felt like an outcast. Race was a large part of the problem. It was not until high school that I felt better socially. That particular school was more diverse than the middle school. Therefore, it was not until high school that I made friends with whom I could relate to.

I loved learning and relished the opportunity to expand my knowledge. However, there was one thing about her school that troubled her deeply—the segregated cafeteria.

Life Support

By and by, I make my way.

It is a mental struggle every day.

Optimism, positivity, strength, and faith I possess, to ease this battle I do best.
Friends, family, and providers have my back, as the

viciousness of this illness attacks. Functionality, talents,

motivation have come, to stay and play because I will

never be done. A bright future ahead in this game called

life, only because I was meant to thrive.

I have never claimed any defeat.

From this life, I will never retreat.

There is hope over the horizon, as the shining sun is rising.

Realization

What do you do when you realize that you are alone?

What do you do when you realize that you are second best? What do you do when you have nothing right?

What do you do when your life feels off? You pray.

You say I am grateful for… You smile.

You work.

You help.

You reflect.

You enjoy.

Then, burdens will fall off of your shoulders. Then, God has a path to guide you down.

Then, people gravitate towards your light. Then, there will be no more plight. Recognize that you are whole. Recognize you are loved.

Recognize you are important in the great scheme of life.

Every day I entered the bustling cafeteria at the school, I couldn't help but notice the stark differences in how the students chose to sit. I observed that the cafeteria seemed divided, not by physical barriers but by unseen lines. There were stark divisions that plagued my school.

In one corner of the room, the tables were filled with predominantly white students. They laughed, socialized, and seemed at ease within their group. Their conversations filled the air, but I noticed something peculiar—among the sea of white faces, there were only a few black students, like myself.

In another corner, a smaller group of black students gathered. Their laughter was subdued, their voices hushed. They sat together, united in their shared experiences, discussing life and advocating for change. It was in this corner that I often found solace and familiarity.

I often wondered why there was such a divide within our high school cafeteria. Was it a result of personal choice, societal expectations, or something deeper? As an astute observer, I understood the impact of history on the present. I knew that segregation was a part of America's past, yet here it was, still lingering in my school.

It was not until high school that I felt better socially. That particular school was more diverse than the middle school. Therefore, it was not until high school that I made friends with whom I could relate to. When I went to boarding school, I found myself immersed in an even more diverse and multicultural environment. It was a great relief to be in such a stimulating and enriching place. I was really lucky to have had that experience.

Stratford Mount Vernon School was a good experience for me in hindsight. Boarding school gave me a certain independence. It taught me a lot about myself and how I relate to certain people and situations.

My trust in people lessened at SMV because of my experience in my old school. I came in contact with a lot of people different from myself from all over the country and around the world. I should have taken the opportunity to get to know people better. However, I did not let people in, even when they welcomed me and reached out to me. I made friends, most of whom I did not keep in contact with. The friendships I maintain from boarding school are little, however they mean a lot to me. I still keep in touch with a set of twins, Natasha and Yolanda Yeboah. They reside in Harlem, NY, and attend Columbia and Amerhest, respectively. They are bright, kind, and a lot of fun. We hung out back in school a lot. Another friend from SMV is Nina Savario. Nina and I were close in our senior year. She went off to Wheaton with me. She comes from Far Rockaway, Queens, but was originally from Jamaica. I am gradually learning how to trust her and be close with her. Sondra Eva was another friend of mine at SMW. She is originally from Colombia. I can honestly say all of these girls are my friends. While I was in boarding school, my family and I were going through a lot with my brother Amaadi. He has special needs; therefore, his behavior was not equal to the outward teenage aggression he exhibited back then. My father took all of this hard. My mother remained strong with all of this, especially outwardly. At school, I felt pressure to succeed for my parents' approval and love. I felt compelled to prove myself to everyone around me but myself. I recall that during the last term of high school, my Mom and Dad aided me in my schoolwork because I was unable to focus. My mind was on all the negative thoughts and happenings of my life at the time. I was not doing my schoolwork, nor did I want to go off to college right away. I felt that I needed a break for a year before going off to Wheaton University. I remember going to the school psychologist in order to rid my record of absence points from the classes I did not attend. Our sessions soon became a different topic. The school psychologist told me that I was mildly depressed. Graduation day came, and I was not engaged in the glee and activities of my classmates. My high school graduation was the worst day of my life. I was miserable, and I did not know completely why. Thankfully, my family and guests did not even see me walk across the stage, except for my mom and dad. It was a mess in my mind, but a glorious occasion for my family and friends. That summer, we all visited a family therapist to discuss the family and the family related to Amaadi. It was helpful to a certain extent. A lot was brought up for open discussion. In the end, Amaadi was to be given professional help on a daily basis. I was convinced, as was the family, that I needed to seek professional help on my own for my needs. Eventually, I saw Dr. Epstein for evaluation and meds before I set off to college. He put me on an antidepressant, Celexa, without a mood stabilizer. This was a grave mistake. The Celexa pushed me into an elevated, euphoric mood by the time I drove off to Wheaton that Fall, an elevated mood that I could not come down from until one month later. The day I came home from school, I was a different person. I was psychotic and delusional. The next day, I went off to a mental health hospital called Bennington Memorial Hospital. I was treated there for psychotic disorder NOS and a rule-out of bipolar illness. I came out of the hospital refreshed, informed, and healthier.

Here were some entries from my senior year of high school:

March 30, 2001:

What's going on right now? I'm listening to some Jill Scott. Track 3. I feel healthy. I feel good. I feel clear. I feel alone, but not really, because I know that I can be upstairs chilling with Nikki or on the phone with someone who likes me. I do enjoy my own company. It's like I know myself, but not really because one, I do not take care of myself, and two, I get shocked at things sometimes.

"Let's take/ a long walk/ around the park/ after dark..." —*Jill Scott*

April 2001: Why Mrs. Rowsey is upset:

O *She thinks I am not putting effort into her class*

O *Can't afford to be late/ absent again or miss the bus*

O *Late 3x's due to bus and today*

O *HW, test case study*

O *No effort in bus today*

O *SWE, workjob, PE, choir, Bio/ Rel, late 1 hr for English*

O *Bio/ Rel o Bus 1 o Bus 1 ❼ late o Today 1*

    o *30-minute late to class because of 8:30 bus*

O *English o Last Thurs. 1 peer auditing*

    o *Late today*

        ☒ *Journal incident*

        ☒ *No vocab word*

        ☒ *Topic for essay*

May 19, 2001:

I was feeling like shit a minute ago until I read all of these past entries. They are really depressing. When I stepped back mentally for a minute and read these entries. I realize the situation I am in. I am depressed... My depression is surrounded by these factors: family, friends, and self. I am crying now. I am sad. Destiny's Child's CD is playing, track number 17, a gospel medley. Someone's calling.

It was Annette. She told me about how my teachers were concerned about me. They feel like I am avoiding things. She says don't be afraid to ask for help. Don't try to do everything on my own. She knows that I am taking medication. I really hope that she doesn't go blabbing about it. I shouldn't have told her. She said something weird. Mrs. Rowsey supposedly thinks that I am avoiding doing the work because of lateness. I am not going to class because I am not doing the work. She told Annette my flies had died. I guess she is trying to say that I am making excuses for not doing my work. She also talked about speaking with Mrs. Brooks about me, saying that Mr. Brooks is concerned about me, and that he does not know what to do. She, Annette, is way too comfortable talking about my business, i.e., BU, telling Angie that and Chris finding out, and then talking to Mrs. Brooks, and now she knows that I'm on meds rather than worry about her telling people, I need to tell her not to share that with anyone. I probably, no, I definitely should have been honest with Annette. She is the only link between me and my teachers, besides my own communication with them. I am in a hole. A very, very deep one.

May 24, 2001:

This is part of the message that I got from my Dad today:
"Dean Faculty has called. It's embarrassing. What is going on? Everybody in my school is worried about this behavior. We can't give any excuse; we can't use depression; we can't use any other excuse for this problem. Finish the paper. May God bless you."

June 1, 2001:

It's the last day of school. I am both going home and graduating in two days. It is just too much for me. My teachers for Genetics and Ethical Decisions basically fucked me over on my paper and presentation. I need to be really productive right now just so I do not find myself in a bind at the last minute. My feelings of agony aside, I have to be productive. I am telling myself to suck it up, in other words.

But, it was not how it seemed on the outside. I was sad and angry and felt very much alone. I remember being one of the only high school seniors who was not excited at the prospect of going away to college the next year. I remember the months leading to the end of my senior year in high school. Stress was a mainstay in my life. I was always seeking perfection. I kept my emotions, worries, and concerns to myself. All the anger I held at the world reversed and bombarded my core. I was gradually becoming depressed. I almost did not finish my college applications because I felt emotionally unprepared to begin such a new and major part of my life. Thankfully, I had the support of my family, and I was able to complete my college applications. Later, I was accepted into four very good schools.

A counselor at my high school diagnosed me with depression, and a doctor began treating me for the illness.

CHAPTER 3:

ME

I am a child of God first and foremost. I am of Ghanaian descent. I have a lot of pride in my African culture. I have been blessed with parents who shared our heritage with my siblings and me. I have been exposed to the language, the food, the music, and other aspects of the Ghanaian way of life. I have traveled to Ghana many times. In general, traveling is a pastime my family and I enjoy.

I dream. I write. I love. I sing. I dance. I have been a dreamer, a writer, and a lover of God all of my life. God is the first and the last being I speak to every day. I would not be here if it were not for Him. My parents exposed my siblings and me to faith. However, God became real to me on a personal level at a very early age. I have always been a prayerful person. However, it was not until age 18 that I fully devoted my life to God.

I am truly in touch with my emotions, and I feel very deeply. I am sensitive. I empathize with the downtrodden and destitute. I have always been that way. My younger brother Amaadi has inspired me to be this way. Only a year-and-a-half separate the two of us. He has taught me so much. I appreciate so much in life because of him. Because he cannot do the simplest things, it makes me grateful to have intellect and ability. I thank God every day for my brother. Amaadi has opened my eyes to the fact that life is a gift.

I am a reporter by training and an observer by birth. I revel in observing what some may see as mundane. I find beauty in the weirdest places. I am a very creative person. Since the age of 10, I have expressed myself through verse. I love writing poetry. My imagination and my dreams have always been immense and endless as the sky up above. I love to dream. My dreams are expressed through my creative writing. Music is another passion of mine. I listen to everything: gospel, R&B, reggae, Latin, African, and rock. I sing in a band at my church. Singing has been a passion of mine since high school. I also love to dance, and I do it every chance that I get.

I share all of this to say, human beings tend to live in an insular way. By sharing our stories, we can create the blueprint to help facilitate the healing of others. While experiencing depression, I was isolated. I gradually learned how to share my story, which, I hope, made a difference in the lives of those with whom I shared.

Aside from my parents, Amaadi has inspired me to pursue my goals. We are close in age, and as a child, I remember feeling a sense of obligation to protect him from the outside world. He has taught me so much. I appreciate life because of him. Because he cannot do the simplest things, it makes me grateful to have intellect and ability. Amaadi has opened my eyes to the fact that life is a gift meant to be shared. He had a strong influence on my decision to become a mental health advocate. In retrospect, I realize I have benefited from growing up with a brother with special needs. His influence has helped me develop patience, empathy, and a passion for aiding the destitute and downtrodden. Our childhood built character and strength in me, which I have applied to my work in public service.

As Ralph Waldo Emerson said, "What lies behind us, what lies before us, are tiny matters compared to what lies within us." I want to empower others who have been through similar experiences as my family. I want our story to be a testament to survival and perseverance to others. All people should strive to be citizens of the world rather than live in an insular, self-serving environment. Not only do we have purposes to fulfill individually, we are also accountable for one another, a responsibility that is bigger than us. Social work and health policy are my interests. I feel an obligation to put something back into the community. I feel that I can make a difference as a member of society and in my professional work. It is my will to continue the legacy of my parents and fight for others in whom I believe, dedicating my life to service and working hard at worthy causes.

I had an onset of depression at the age of 17. I overcame depression for a period of 13 years, primarily dealing with the symptoms of anxiety during that time. I remember the months leading to the end of my senior year in high school.

I was sad and angry, and I felt very much alone. Stress was a mainstay in my life. I kept my emotions, worries, and concerns to myself. I was gradually becoming depressed.

I managed to start my freshman year of college feeling optimistic, but depression was still hiding in the shadows. I found myself socializing a lot, sleeping very little, and studying even less. I was on a downward spiral, which ended in a severe emotional crash or breakdown. I had to take a medical leave of absence from my school.

By the start of my freshman year at Wilmington University, I was in fairly good spirits. I felt, so I thought, strong enough to begin my college career. Unbeknownst to me, I was experiencing an unnatural high, something I never experienced again until my later 30s.

These symptoms of hypomania and mania were a shock to my system that I thankfully overcame. In theory, the medication I was on had put me in an elevated mood. I found myself socializing a lot, sleeping very little, and studying even less. I was on a downward spiral, which ended in a severe emotional crash or breakdown. I had to take a medical leave of absence from my school, and I was admitted to a psychiatric hospital for a psychotic break at the age of 18. I was eventually stabilized and discharged from the hospital.

CHAPTER 4:

SHARING, STORYTELLING AND ADVOCACY – MENTAL HEALTH AND COPING

That time marked the beginning of a life of medication, titration, counseling, and treatment goals. I took classes part-time as I was working on remaining stable. This meant that aside from working towards a degree, I was looking for medical providers, as well as a medicine regimen that worked best for me.

That period in time was also a very trying, uplifting, and eye-opening experience for my family and me, all wrapped in one. Life was different after the second hospital discharge because I finally found caring and skilled medical providers, as well as the right medication and a clearer diagnosis. In addition, I had the continued support of my family.

In my 20s, I waffled back and forth between anxiety and healing. I identified with the Book of Job. I felt like I went through a lot in the past, and I was being punished. Yet, my faith in God persisted. I lived the quote, "The Lord didn't promise that life would be easy, but He did promise to go with you every step of the way."

When in difficulty, do not ask for faithfulness. Rather, no matter what happens, you are still faithful, which does not necessarily mean God will not let something challenging happen. Even when doing everything right, you can still go through it. God said, you can touch her, Satan, but you cannot touch her soul. No matter what you do, you will not succeed. I learned, in those years, that God is real! I also learned to take God's Word literally and not doubt it.

My 20s were a time of prayer, reading God's Word, witnessing, eating better, working out again, branching out socially, medication compliance, getting help with my anxiety through excellent providers, and networking.

September 22, 2010: A letter to my Father:

Dear God,

I love you. We have been down a very long and difficult road together. Thank you so much. The old is gone. The new is here. I have been through so much, but you took me out and gave me strength to continue. Lord, my past is full of so much pain. I have been bruised and battered, but I am not broken. Thank you so much. Harassment at Brooklawn School. I remember it all. But look at me now. People look up to me now.

Abba! Thank you. I love You. I am using that pain to help younger kids. Kenya is an example. Kenya, as you know, is a student at MS 203 in the Bronx (New York). She is constantly bullied. She has low self-esteem. God, help her. I realize that my past experiences can be used in my work as a social worker. I can empower young girls. I have been through so much stress and anxiety growing up in the Adade household. It was rough.

Amaadi, the love of my life, and my favorite sibling, Abba, please keep him and watch over him and let him know he is always loved—Amaadi's existence is a blessing. However, the stress of his care has taken a toll on the whole family. It has also caused a divide in Mom and Dad's relationship. These dynamics and more created a chaotic home life. I have suffered from extreme anxiety and constant stress because of it.

But the old is gone; the new is here. There have been positive people and experiences in my life. I am blessed. Continuing from my previous dialogue, I have also experienced trauma. Four Sails Hospital. That was a very dark, difficult place. Abba, thank you! I survived. It was so hard being a patient in a psychiatric hospital. But, I have lived to tell the story. For that, Lord, I am grateful. Though I have had numerous panic attacks, breakdowns, and conversion disorder symptoms, I am sane. Thank you. It was all for a reason.

I have helped people who suffer from mental illness. Look at my work at the NAMI. I have helped NAMI members through my story and my testimony. I have given the mentally ill a voice. I have put their plight in the ears of legislators—literally. Wow! Yes, me. Andrea Anastasia Andrews. The girl who used to be shy, depressed, and defeated has dedicated her life to serving others. I made it. Father, I know you already know because you are the Creator of the universe and Maker of Heaven and Earth. You are the chief designer and orchestrator of my life. Thank you. Father, I am free! Everything happened for a reason."

I had a passion for helping children overcome their challenges. My first-year field placement was in the South Bronx of New York. I believed in the power of group therapy to bring about positive change.

One day, as I walked through the doors of MS 203, I sensed a palpable aura of tension and frustration resonating throughout the hallways.

Us social work interns had a comfortable and inviting office. Kenya, a 13-year-old girl, sat nervously in a chair across from me. She had been experiencing constant bullying at school, which had caused her self-esteem to plummet.

"Good morning, Kenya. I'm glad you could make it today. How are you feeling?"

"I'm feeling alright, I guess. The bullying at school has been really tough though. I don't know what to do anymore."

"I understand how challenging this must be for you, Kenya. You don't deserve to be mistreated, and it's important to work through these emotions together. Can you tell me more about what's been happening?"

"Well, it started a few months ago. There's this group of girls who keep making fun of me, calling me names, and spreading rumors about me. It's made me feel so small and worthless. It's hard for me to believe in myself anymore."

"I'm really sorry to hear that, Kenya. You are none of the things they're saying about you. You are a remarkable person with many strengths and talents. It's understandable that their hurtful words have affected your self-esteem, but we can work on building it back up.

What are some things you like about yourself?"

She paused. "Well, I really enjoy drawing in my sketchbook. I think I'm pretty good at it. And I'm also a good listener. People often come to me for advice."

"That's wonderful to hear, Kenya. Those are excellent qualities. It's important to recognize and appreciate your own gifts and talents. We can focus on enhancing your self-esteem by nurturing those strengths.

How does that sound to you?"

"I think it could help. I just wish things would get better at school."

"Let's work together to make that happen, Kenya. Firstly, I want to assure you that you are not alone in this. It's never easy dealing with bullying, but there are steps we can take to address the situation. Have you spoken to any teachers or the school counselor about what's been going on?"

"I haven't yet. I'm just afraid it will make things worse if the bullies find out."

"I understand your concerns, Kenya. It's important to prioritize your safety and well-being. However, it's also crucial that the adults at school are aware of the issue, as they can provide support and help put a stop to bullying. Together, we can come up with a plan that ensures your safety and involves trusted adults."

"Okay, I'll consider talking to someone about it."

"That's a great step forward, Kenya. Remember, you deserve to be treated with respect, and we will work on strategies to encourage positive interactions with your peers. In the meantime, let's focus on building your self-esteem and finding healthy coping mechanisms to deal with the negative emotions you've been experiencing. Does that sound good to you?"

"Yes, that sounds like a good plan, Ms. Andrea. I really appreciate your help."

"It's my pleasure to assist you, Kenya. Remember, you are strong, talented, and deserving of kindness. We'll work through this together, step by step. Is there anything else you'd like to share or discuss today?"

"Not right now, but thank you again, Ms. Andrea. I'm glad I have someone to talk to who understands."

"Anytime, Kenya. I'm here to support you. We'll schedule our next session soon, and until then, remember to be kind to yourself. You're doing great."

Kenya nodded, with a hint of a smile appearing as hope began to shine through her eyes.

Concerned about the well-being of the students, I decided to start an anger management group at the school. I believed that by teaching the students healthy ways to express and manage their anger, I could create a safer and more harmonious environment for everyone. With the support of the school's principal and staff, I set out to make a difference.

I gathered a diverse group of middle schoolers who were struggling with anger issues. There was Michael, an intense and fiery boy who had trouble controlling his temper. Sarah, a quiet girl with a lot of pent-up frustration, often found herself bottling up her emotions until she exploded. And then there was Ethan, a volatile student who tended to resort to physical aggression when overwhelmed. I knew that reaching out to these students and others like them was crucial for their personal growth.

The first day of the group arrived, and I began by creating a safe and non-judgmental environment. I reminded the students that anger was a natural emotion, but it was important to find healthy outlets for it. I asked each student to share their personal experiences with anger, creating a space for open and honest conversation.

As the weeks went by, I introduced various coping mechanisms and emotional regulation techniques. I taught the students how to identify triggers, practice deep breathing exercises, and use positive self-talk to manage their anger. The group engaged in role-playing activities, where they learned to communicate assertively and express their needs and feelings without resorting to aggression.

I also recognized the importance of fostering empathy among the students. I organized activities that encouraged them to put themselves in each other's shoes and understand the potential impact of their actions on others. Through these exercises, Michael, Sarah, and Ethan realized that their anger was often a response to their own internal struggles and that finding healthy coping mechanisms was crucial for their growth.

Over time, the anger management group became a safe haven for the students, a place where they felt heard and understood. They began to form lasting friendships, supporting each other through their anger challenges. The once tense hallways of MS 203 slowly transformed into a more peaceful environment.

I knew that my work was far from over, but I had seen the transformation I had hoped for. The students were now equipped with the tools to recognize and manage their anger, empowering them to make healthier choices in their lives. As I bid farewell to her middle school group, I felt a sense of fulfillment knowing that

Once upon a time, in the bustling city of Bronxville, there was a renowned psychiatrist named Dr. Hasan Asif. Dr. Asif had dedicated his life to helping people overcome their mental struggles and find inner peace. His reputation for exceptional listening skills and compassion had made him one of the most sought-after psychiatrists in the area. One of Dr. Asif's long-time clients was me. I had been battling anxiety and depression for as long as I could remember. I had tried various therapies and medications, but nothing seemed to offer me lasting relief.

I remember our first meeting. It was a darkish room with windows high up, shaded with blue curtains. He asked me basic questions. But, I was only a quarter of the way listening. My brain was overwhelmed by the group session we just had at the outpatient facility. So, I answered "yes" to every question. Who knew that this meeting would be the catalyst for a positive, educational, and extremely helpful therapeutic relationship? I owe seeing myself as more than a diagnosis, having a clear diagnosis and appropriate and effective medication to Dr. Hasan Asif.

Our sessions started with Dr. Asif asking gentle questions to understand my experiences and emotions better. I, initially hesitant and guarded, gradually opened up, trusting his expertise. Our conversations flowed seamlessly between discussion and dialogue.

"Good morning, Andrea," Dr. Asif said. "How have you been since our last session?"

I said, "Honestly, it's been a rollercoaster. Some days are better than others, but overall, I still feel overwhelmed by my thoughts and worries."

"I appreciate your honesty, Andrea," he responded. "Let's delve into the root causes of your anxiety and depression. Can you recall any specific triggers or events that have recently affected your mental well-being?"

"Well, I've been struggling with self-doubt and feelings of inadequacy at work. It seems no matter how hard I try, I can never reach the expectations I set for myself. It's frustrating, and it takes a toll on my self-esteem."

Dr. Asif said, "It's important to acknowledge that you're not alone in feeling this way, Andrea. Many people face similar challenges. Let's explore ways to manage these expectations and build confidence in your abilities. Have you considered any self-care practices or relaxation techniques?"

I said, "I've tried a few things, like exercise, but I struggle to consistently incorporate them into my routine. I guess I feel guilty for taking time for myself when I could be working or doing something productive."

Dr. Asif responded, "Andrea, self-care isn't selfish or unproductive. It's crucial for maintaining mental well-being and giving yourself the care you deserve. We'll work together to find the right balance. Let's devise a plan that includes self-care activities you genuinely enjoy."

As the sessions continued, Dr. Asif guided me towards gradually implementing self-care practices. Together, we explored different techniques until they found ones that resonated with my personality and interests. Dr. Asif also encouraged me to challenge my negative thoughts and reframe them into more positive and realistic beliefs.

Months passed, and I started to notice positive changes in my life. My anxiety began to ebb away, and with Dr. Asif's guidance, I gained a sense of control over my emotions. My newfound confidence not only led to improvements in my professional life but also deepened my personal relationships.

Dr. Asif, witnessing my ongoing growth and transformation, couldn't help but feel immense satisfaction in his role as a guide and healer. He knew that his purpose was to create a safe space for his clients, helping them navigate their mental landscapes and find their own paths towards happiness and fulfillment.

Make Me Over
Stagnant in a season of abundance.
The man with the one talent I do not want to be. A heart
full of gratitude, a spirit full of joy, because of what my
heavenly Father has done for me.
I am walking in freedom.
The shackles have been broken for some time now.
Despite this season of increase, my heart feels gray at times. My spirit
feels laden with sorrow at times.

Guilt, shame, fear, and trembling occupy space within me, space that belongs to joy.

In this season of multiple blessings, I pray, God, make me over.

Make me into a vessel that shouts hallelujahs and sweet hymns of praise for what my God has done for me. I am tired of messing up time after time, especially as I thrive in this season of unmerited favor.

Father, any way about me that is not of You, take it away.

Give me the strength I need to change.

No more stagnation.

No more burying talents.

No more sorrow.

No more guilt and shame.

No more fear and trembling.

Make me over, Father.

My heart's desire is to be the new creation you have made me.

Thank you for your forgiveness, Father.

Thank you for your favor, Father, You are amazing.

You brought me through many trials and tribulations.

I am still alive and well because of You, Father.

I am already made over, with a new spirit, and it is because of you, Father. Take away all and everything that separates me from You, so that I may spend eternity with You.

It is all yours, Father, I am here on bended knees, with my arms outstretched, in full surrender to You, Father. Thank you for this season and the many seasons that will come my way.

My Mom prays with and for me every day. Sometimes, I do not even have to give her a prayer request, but she accurately prays for exactly what I need. I have a select few friends with this gift who I pray and fast with.

One evening, as the setting sun cast a warm glow through the window, I heard a knock on my apartment door. To my disbelief, it was my Mom. She traveled all the way from Connecticut via train, no doubt since she hated driving on the highway. She looked worried and tired. I said, "Come in." We sat together, our hands clasped tightly in prayer.

"Dear God, thank you for this day and for the many blessings you have given us. Please watch over our family and guide us through any challenges we may face. Amen."

"Amen. Andrea, my dear, I'm so grateful for your unwavering faith and that we can come to God together to find strength and support. Remember, no matter what, you are never alone." I cherished these moments of connection, where we shared our hopes and fears with one another and sought solace in our faith.

As the weeks went on, my life presented me with both joyous moments and difficult obstacles. Through it all, my Mom remained a steadfast pillar of support. One afternoon, after a particularly challenging day at school, I came home feeling defeated and deflated. My Mom, sensing her daughter's distress, welcomed her with open arms.

It reminded her of a conversation we had during my freshman year of high school.

"Mom, I don't understand why some kids at school are being mean to me for no reason. It hurts, and it makes me question myself."

"Oh, my precious girl, I'm sorry you have had to face such unkindness," she stated. "Remember, people's behavior often stems from their own insecurities and struggles. What matters is how you respond. Let's talk about some ways to navigate these difficult situations and rise above the negativity."

The two of us spent the evening talking, laughing, and coming up with practical solutions to address the challenges I faced at school. My Mom's unwavering love and support helped me feel empowered and ready to face whatever came my way.

CHAPTER 5:

MENTAL HEALTH AND ADVOCACY

I am a walking miracle. God showed me the way. I am a walking miracle. It is a new day!

Over time, my confidence soared, and my resilience grew stronger. As I faced new challenges, I knew I could turn to prayer and my mother's wisdom for guidance and strength. Our bond deepened, and together, we formed an unbreakable support system.

In the years that followed grad school, I went on to achieve remarkable success in many aspects of my life. But what remained constant was my unwavering connection to my faith and my mother's unending love. My Mom is special to me. I remember the silky smooth feel of her morning gown between my fingers as I followed her like a duckling to the kitchen stove, where the aroma of pancakes, eggs, and sausage filled the air every Sunday morning before church. I remember the birthday parties at Chi Chi's with Notes the Clown, making balloon animals. My Mom is a rare woman, a uniquely crafted jewel created in God's image. She is an everywoman—hard-working and successful. She is a pillar of faith and fortitude. She is spiritually sound. I thank her for her unceasing prayers for her loved ones. Her beauty is inside and out. She commands attention everywhere she goes. My Mom carries herself with boldness and confidence. She is intelligent with a master's degree in Food Science and Industrial Microbiology. Her wisdom is unending. She is generous, always serving others. The world is brighter and better with her.

Her way of dealing with our familial problems is to not deal with them. She becomes overwhelmed, and then she shuts down. Mom has many physical ailments. She needs help with my brother, Amaadi, with the house, and for herself so she does not break apart emotionally and physically. She got in a car accident in November last year. This changed her perspective greatly. She saw that her job took a large toll on her physically and mentally. She discovered that she needed extra time for herself. I love my mother, and I worry about her. She goes through a lot of stress daily, as well as constant pain.

In a brightly lit auditorium, a diverse audience gathered, eager to listen and learn about mental health. A stage adorned with a simple podium stood in the center, ready to host a powerful conversation. It was a National Alliance on Mental Illness Connecticut conference. Among the attendees was me, a courageous young woman who had embarked on a journey of self-discovery and healing. As the moderator introduced me, I stepped forward, took a deep breath, and began to share my story.

"Good evening, everyone," I said. "Thank you for being here. As someone who has struggled with mental health, I believe it's crucial to break the silence and create a safe space for dialogue. My journey has been difficult, but I am here today to remind you that there is hope, no matter how dark things may seem."

The audience listened attentively, their eyes fixed upon me, ready to absorb my words.

Growing up, I always felt like an outsider, with anxiety and depression, whispering in my ear that I wasn't good enough. That is where my focus was. I battled my demons in silence, afraid of judgment and stigma. But one day, I realized that I couldn't let those fears control me any longer.

I paused, my voice wavering slightly with emotion, but my determination shone through.

"Seeking help was one of the scariest yet most empowering decisions I've ever made. I found a psychiatrist who became my guide and partner in this journey. He taught me that my struggles didn't define me and that it was okay to feel vulnerable. Through therapy, I learned to lean on my support system, and gradually, I began to heal.

A murmur of support rippled through the audience as they connected with my heartfelt words.

I continued, "But the healing didn't end with therapy alone. I discovered the power of self-care, of nurturing my mind and body. Meditation and engaging in activities I love became my lifelines. I realized the importance of setting boundaries and taking time to nurture my own well-being."

The audience nodded, affirming the wisdom and importance of self-care.

"Education played a vital role in my journey as well," I said. "I devoured books and articles to understand my own mind better. By learning about different mental health conditions, I not only gained insight into my struggles but also found compassion for others who may be walking a similar path."

A woman in the front row wiped away a tear, as if my story had touched something deep within her own experience.

I continued, "Today, my goal is to advocate for mental health awareness and change the narrative surrounding it. Let's encourage a culture of understanding and empathy. Let's be the support system that someone else might desperately need." The audience erupted into applause, their genuine appreciation filling the air. My vulnerability and strength had resonated with them deeply.

As I stepped back from the podium, I felt a sense of pride, knowing that my story had touched the hearts of many. I had taken the first step—sharing my truth—and now, I knew I wasn't alone in my journey towards mental well-being.

Act 2:

Inside Me
Inside me is a story, a story of
love.
You will find my God, alive, on
fire, in my heart. Inside me is a
book, with many chapters
untouched.
On these words, emotions, and fantasies, I have a
clutch. Inside me is a river that flows to no end.
Passion runs through it, and vigor roars at every bend.
Inside me are questions, some answered, some not, a
collection of deep inferences I have never forgotten, that
in finality will be deduced. Inside me is a deep
mourning,
for all the parts of my decadent moments of joy,
a mourning, replaced with poinsettias, which blossom, and
I feel. Inside me are conflictions, one about my birth
brother and one about my wings. Conflictions that burn,
when the venom of choices and non-choices sting. Inside me
are fears, fears about worries, and worries about fears.
These circles bring abundant tears.
Inside me is perfect peace.
Nothing is new, fledging is an old pastime. Shiny stars
illuminate my interior, until my interior rises up and up farther
into the layers of the sun.

I am a firm believer that all things happen for a reason. It is not a mistake that I, a young journalist with a bachelor's degree in English, discovered a passion for social work. My career in journalism began in high school, where I wrote for the school newspaper. During my college years, I wrote for the campus newspaper and completed internships at community publications. After college, I became the sole full-time reporter at the Fairfield (CT) Minuteman Newspaper. I am a leader and a people-oriented person, traits that helped me succeed as a reporter. The best experiences I have had in journalism were performing the basic tasks of interviewing people from different walks of life. Journalism has taught me that everyone has a story.

While I pursued a career in journalism, I remained active within my community through volunteerism. As a teenager, I served as a volunteer with the Stamford (CT) Hospital Bennett Cancer Walk and St. Luke's LifeWorks, a Connecticut-based organization that provides programs that serve individuals affected by homelessness, HIV/AIDS, and mental illness. In my senior year of high school, I worked at a women's shelter, the New England Learning Center for Women in Transition, in Greenfield, Massachusetts. I recently completed an internship with the Stamford (CT) Health Department. My work at the Stamford Health Department involved rotations in all divisions of the department, namely HIV Prevention and the Stamford Health Department STD clinic.

My interest in a new career began when I joined the National Alliance on Mental Illness (NAMI) Fairfield, Connecticut, chapter while pursuing my undergraduate degree in English. NAMI is the nation's largest grassroots health organization dedicated to improving the lives of people with serious mental illnesses and their families. I am passionate about mental health advocacy and the fight for mental health parity. I am also an active member of the

NAMI Fairfield Board of Directors. My participation in NAMI changed my life. I have identified my strong desire to make an impact on mental health parity through public policy that will positively impact those affected by mental disabilities.

Traits that set me apart from others are my strong empathy and compassion for others, as well as my drive and commitment. An example of the distance I am willing to travel for others is the leadership role I assumed when I became the liaison between NAMI Fairfield and NAMI on Campus Fairfield University, an affiliate of the national organization. It is a student-run organization designed to educate campus communities about mental illness while promoting early detection and intervention and fighting the stigma surrounding mental illnesses. I created the group because I knew the importance of making an organization such as NAMI on Campus available to students. There is a large stigma surrounding mental illnesses, which are not recognized as brain disorders. Mental illness is a reality for many college students, and three-quarters of all lifetime cases of mental illness begin by age 24.[1] I wanted to bring both awareness of mental illness to my school and support to my fellow students who needed the service.

Starting and maintaining NAMI on Campus at Fairfield University was a large commitment and a difficult task. Becoming an official NAMI on Campus group required endorsement by both the local and state NAMI organizations (NAMI Fairfield and NAMI Connecticut),

---

[1] https://nami.org

approval from NAMI National, and recognition of the university. I ran into many roadblocks as the founder of my school's chapter. To be granted club status by NAMI for my affiliate, I needed a minimum of five organization members. Establishing the on-campus affiliate was a challenge because it was difficult to galvanize an initial group of students equally passionate as I was about forming a mental health advocacy group at our school. I began the initiative as a college senior, another concern because I needed to find a group of underclassmen who could maintain the organization after I graduated from the university.

It was not easy to highlight mental illness at a homogeneous, nondiverse Jesuit institution, where sensitive topics that affect students are not regularly discussed. Major challenges I faced were recruiting members, bringing group members together at meetings, and publicizing the organization. I raised awareness by writing articles in the school newspaper, and making a case for the inception of NAMI on Campus. For example, I wrote an article on the rising statistics of college-aged depression. For a long while, attendance at the first meetings was extremely low, to the extent that on some days, I was the only person present. I did not give up because I knew some people were willing to partake in the initiative. It was a long and arduous process, but I was committed and eventually successfully brought it to fruition.

My recruiting efforts continued after graduation as I worked closely with the President of NAMI Fairfield, a professor at the Fairfield University School of Nursing, and the Director of the Fairfield University counseling services to create an action plan. I dug deep, and finally, before graduation, I identified a dedicated underclassman willing to continue where I left off and serve as President of the campus affiliate. I worked closely with the student, coaching and supporting her as the organization grew. We increased membership and visibility by organizing activities, such as movie nights, which featured films with mental health themes. We created announcements on the campus-wide email system, posted flyers around the school, and publicized the group at the university health fair. I organized local media coverage, and as a reporter for a major town newspaper, I wrote about the initiative in local publications.

From start to finish, it took a total of two years to make NAMI on Campus Fairfield University the thriving success it is today. It took time for the group to attain recognition by the university administration as an official student organization. After the university's decision, the wait continued as the campus affiliate went through the NAMI National chartering process.

NAMI on Campus Fairfield University is now the second university affiliate to be established in the state of Connecticut.

I also had the privilege of serving as Liaison in Strategic Partnerships and coordinated the planning of the NAMI Fairfield annual legislative social with board members, as well as federal and local legislators in mental health agencies, to discuss mental health parity health care access, supportive housing, young adult services, school-based services, mental community health services, legislative funding, and cost-effective solutions that enable life and recovery with mental illness.

CHAPTER 6:

MENTAL HEALTH AND PUBLIC HEALTH

Affordable and accessible health care is a right, not an option. In this economic climate, millions of Americans are uninsured, and just as many are at risk of losing their insurance. According to health statistics, more than one in four uninsured adults has a mental illness and/or substance abuse disorder.[2] Many states do not have public health insurance plans that proficiently meet the needs of Americans with mental illness, even though 46 percent of Americans will meet the criteria for a diagnosable mental health condition sometime in their life, and half of those people will develop conditions by the age of 14.[3] Nearly one in five American adults will have a diagnosable mental health condition in any given year.[4] Forty-four million, or 18 percent of, U.S. adults have a mental illness.[5] One in five U.S.

---

[2] https://nami.org
[3] www.mhanational.org
[4] www.mhanational.org
[5] www.mhanational.org

adults experiences mental illness each year.[6] One in twenty U.S. adults experiences serious mental illness each year.[7] One in six U.S. youth aged 6–17 experience a mental health disorder each year. [8]

There is a need for a national health care policy that provides the uninsured the opportunity to improve their health with the support of a federal plan that holds insurance companies accountable. Those without health insurance should have the option of new, affordable health insurance options and a plan that allows them access to affordable health coverage. An improved health policy is important because it can create a high-quality national mental health care system.

I frequently encounter NAMI members who are uninsured and cannot afford proper care. Often, they fall through the cracks of the health care system because of inadequate services. It lowers their morale and leads to untreated illnesses. People living with these serious mental disorders often do not receive adequate services and support. NAMI members who participate in support groups or peer education sessions often report the burdensome out-of-pocket expense of necessary treatment. It is quite devastating to witness a family or individuals who cannot afford treatment for their illnesses or suffer a relapse in their symptoms because their illness goes untreated. All too often, these circumstances have negative effects on their long-term health. This phenomenon also leads to overburdened

---

[6] https://nami.org
[7] https://nami.org
[8] https://nami.org

emergency departments, hospital wards, and public systems. I am passionate about this issue because it is the story of so many.

Mental health services often receive inadequate funding because of poor financing at the state level. A significant number of states do not provide or finance core mental health treatment and recovery services, seek parity in insurance coverage for mental health disorders, provide adequate support to the mentally ill and their families, nor collect and utilize sufficient data on essential mental health services.

Resources exist to properly treat and support Americans who are mentally ill; however, stigma, among other factors, prevents our fellow citizens from leading functional lives and contributing to society. Governors and state legislators in Washington have the authority to turn these circumstances around by providing more support to state mental health agencies, which struggle to provide basic services to the seriously ill. Valiant efforts have been made; however, there is room for improvement.

I never thought that I would end up at a premier school for social work, let alone the only Ivy League one. I am a strong believer that all things happen for a reason. Chance did not bring me into this field. At Crayton, I conducted weekly individual mental health counseling sessions with ten middle school students regarding academic and behavioral challenges. I collaborated with teachers, paraprofessionals, and resource aids to create specific goals and behavior plans for the students, assessed the needs of families via home visits, and facilitated anger management and bereavement group counseling sessions at MS 203 in the South Bronx of New York.

There is always a light at the end of the tunnel, and nothing happens by chance. There were times during my depression and experiences with anxiety I thought God did not love me. I realized later He was setting me up for greatness. Everything in life happens for a reason. Our individual stories can be the blueprint for someone else's healing, meaning we can turn our pain into a tool that can make a difference in this world. I encourage you, reader, to share your story. You can save a life with your hardships. God does not put us through pain to make us suffer. Rather, He wants us to use our stories to help other people.

That time marked the beginning of a life of medication, titration, counseling, and treatment goals. I took classes part-time as I was working on remaining stable. This meant that aside from working towards a degree, I was looking for medical providers, as well as a medicine regimen that worked best for me. The confusion and stress of piecing my life back together and lack of compliance with medication led to a second breakdown and a second hospitalization at the age of 19.

That period in time was a very trying, uplifting, and eye-opening experience for my family and me, all wrapped in one. Life was different after the second hospital discharge because I finally found caring and skilled medical providers, as well as the right medication and a clearer diagnosis. In addition, I had the continued support of my family.

Today, I am a college graduate and a reporter. I have a bright future in journalism and international affairs, two of my main passions. My recovery from mental illness has been a journey. It was a long road, but I did it. I am now at a place where I am very comfortable with who I am. I owe my recovery to God, my loving and supportive family, loyal friends, skilled medical providers, a clear diagnosis, and appropriate and effective medication.

I have very loving relationships with my family and friends. I have a strong relationship with God. All of them have helped me realize my humanity and that I am more than an illness. It took me a long time to accept my diagnosis. I was ashamed for a long time, to the point where I recoiled away from close friends, keeping my experience a secret because I feared rejection. I also found myself not fully accepting that there was something wrong with me.

I ultimately realized that I had true friends when they continued to accept me for who I was. I have found that the more I accept what has happened to me, the more healing gets done. This acceptance made it easier for me to disclose my struggles with mental illness to friends. It is impossible to fight mental illness on one's own. There were times when I felt that there was no need to disclose all of my concerns to health providers and family members. I felt ashamed, and I feared being labeled crazy. It is so important to be open to other people about critical mental health concerns, especially people who are there to help you.

Being a part of NAMI Fairfield has been life-changing. I intend to be a part of mental health advocacy no matter where life takes me. I want to empower others who have been through similar experiences as me. I want my story to be a testament to survival and perseverance to others.

Stratford Mount Vernon School was a good experience for me in hindsight. Boarding school gave me a certain independence. It taught me a lot about myself and how I relate to certain people and situations.

Mania
By Audrey Adobea Adade

Confusion.
Delusion.
Mistrust.

Acting out,   not figuring out.
Loneliness.
Hopelessness.

Pure fright.
No delight.
Rain and pain.
Disdain.

No tomorrow.

Full of sorrow.
Shaken soul.
No control.

Mania.

I journaled about the experience:

> *Crew was difficult on Wednesday. I was out of it and not sure of myself. My strokes were horrible. I was doubting my strength and mixing it with doubting the strength God gave me. It was a horrible feeling. I now know that doubting my own ability is part of being human. I should not confuse that with doubting God's promises to me. So I went to the Health Center still out of it, and told the nurse eventually that I had not eaten that day and that I wanted to speak with Dr. Coughlin.*

> *I went to the A.M.E. Zion church to pray early in the morning. I was not expecting to see anyone there, but Deborah, the reverend, was there in a prayer session with a member of the church. Mrs. Watson, another member, soon came into the church. I spoke to Deborah about how I had given up all of my burdens to God the day before and how deeply he touched me. I was in a tired, worn-out mood while   in   the   church.*

> *After returning from the church to my dorm, I showered. While showering, I received the Holy Spirit. That morning, I decided that I wanted to be saved. Since I was feeling strange and out of it that afternoon, I decided to contact Deborah again. I called her number but got no response. Eventually, I called Mrs. Watson's number. She was home. I told her that I needed to meet someone, particularly Deborah, at the church right away. She said, "Okay." I did not take Celexa that morning either. So that must have added to the deliriousness. I did go to the Health Center after leaving crew practice (where I left my jacket and keys), still out of it and acting strange.*

So I made my way to the A.M.E. Zion church to be saved as I had decided that morning. Deborah, Mrs. Watson, and another reverend whose name I did not recall, were all there with me at the church. They made sure that I took my day Celexa that night after the whole experience. The rest of my Celexa was in the mailroom at school. My experience getting saved at the A.M.E. Zion church was both a scary and a blessed experience. I am grateful to God for the experience despite the fear that factored into the whole experience. I feel completely happy that I have put God first in my life. And I feel extremely grateful to God for touching me so deeply.

I would not have survived if not for my family, especially my brother, who kept me going. His inspiring me was the strength I needed to get through every day. Whenever I would feel doubtful, I would think about how I needed to be there for him. The same goes for my family. I wanted to be there for them too. They helped me through so much. I owed them. They made sacrifices for me, sacrifices they did not have to make. When you have special people in your life, hold onto them. Remember, you are loved. Also, remember to reciprocate. They did not have to do it. I always think about the encouraging words my parents, in particular, had for me. Those words provided me with hope and strength to continue to another day. I rose because of those words. I became strong because of those words. I felt I could conquer the world because of those words. Those words were the wind beneath my wings. I needed the encouragement because the past was traumatizing. My parents were always loyal to me and never allowed others to degrade me. They were never passive-aggressive. They always gave it to me straight when I was in the wrong. They, at the same time, acknowledged me and congratulated me on my many accomplishments. That is what I needed. I needed to feel seen and heard. Be around people who see you as more than a diagnosis.

CHAPTER 7:

MEDICATION – MENTAL HEALTH AND PHYSICAL HEALTH

The effects of medication can sometimes outweigh its purpose. My medication has affected me in many ways, but the side effects have been, at times, overwhelming. It is like watching an ice skater skating. At first sight, things seem serene and beautiful, in this case, the benefits of taking the medications; but, when you take a closer look, a lot of energy, time, money, and effort is expelled. It is an arduous road.

And then there were the effects of my medication. I felt tired often, which prevented me from being social, particularly when I was feeling depressed. I gained a lot of weight too. So, that meant not being able to fit into clothes. My natural size is a size 8. Yes, due to medications, I went up to a size 16. I loved to dress up. I have been that way since the age of 11. I also enjoyed dressing up when going out. So, when I could not fit into my clothing, it was a huge blow to me. When I was small (my weight fluctuated), I felt confident and in control. When I was large, I had low self-esteem.

Succumb

*My eyes are
slumbering.*

*My heart is a
pumping.*

Time is a ticking.

My own butt I am kicking.

*My mind is manufacturing all sorts of negative thoughts.
These thoughts are turning into extreme doubts.*

*These
doubts have no
place. In me, there is no
space.*

*I will go at my
own healthy pace, in order
to finish this race.*

*I can do it all with my God
by my side. When it becomes
unbearable, I will not hide. I am not
going to succumb, to the pressure that
has come. I won't stop until it's all
done.*

From my responsibilities, I will not run.

I was created to be a conqueror and a soldier for my
Lord. I have a shield of faith and God's truth as my sword.

The Silent Struggle - The alarm clock blares in my ears,
shattering my peaceful slumber. As I drag myself out of bed,
a familiar heaviness settles in my chest, a sense of sorrow that
refuses to dissipate. It's been months since I started
experiencing this unrelenting sadness, and each day feels like

a battle to survive. Today, though, is different. Today, I start my journey with medication.

The Pill Bottles Whisper - As I stand in front of the pharmacy counter, the plethora of pill bottles beckoning me forward, I can't shake the feeling of vulnerability. The weight of my mental illness has left me feeling isolated and disconnected, but these tiny capsules hold the promise of a brighter tomorrow. With trembling hands, I accept the bag filled with hope and uncertainty.

The Dance of Chemistry - At first, the medication is a foreign presence in my body. Its introduction causes a delicate dance of chemistry within me. Adjusting to the side effects and new sensations feels like navigating a labyrinth. Yet, as the days pass, the invisible threads binding my mental health to my physical health begin to intertwine.

The Unraveling - One morning, as rays of sunlight filter through my bedroom window, I notice a subtle shift in my mood. The heaviness that has plagued me for so long seems to lift, like a dark cloud dissipating. The medication, once a stranger, has gently unraveled the tangled knots of my mind, allowing me to glimpse the person I once was, and the person I can be once again.

The Wholeness Within - As the weeks turn into months, the medication becomes an undeniable part of my daily routine. It's not a magic bullet, but rather a key that unlocks the door to a better life. The barriers between mental health and physical health dissolve, revealing a holistic sense of well-being.

The Stigma Erased - Through my journey with medication, I come to realize the powerful role it plays in both mental and physical health. The stigma surrounding medication begins to crumble as I learn to advocate for myself and educate others about the importance of integrating mental health into our overall well-being.

Beyond the Pages - My story is just one of many that illuminate the intersection of mental and physical health. By sharing my experiences, I hope to raise awareness and promote understanding. Together, we can bridge the divide between the two and create a world where medication is not seen as a crutch, but rather a vital tool on the path to healing.

The bustling city streets buzzed with life as I sat in the comfort of my home, surrounded by the gentle hum of conversation and the aroma of freshly brewed coffee. But beneath the surface, an unsettling truth stirred within me—a truth that tested the limits of my belief in the power of medication.

It began innocently enough, with a single pill to alleviate a persistent physical ailment. As the days turned into weeks and then months, I was faced with a sobering reality—I had become a prisoner of medication. What was supposed to offer relief had morphed into a relentless cycle of side effects and dependency.

The Trials of Transformation - The side effects penetrated every aspect of my existence, eroding the sense of self I had once known. The weight gain and appetite fluctuations made me feel like a stranger in my own body, no longer recognizing my reflection in the mirror. Fatigue became my constant companion, enveloping me in a haze of exhaustion that stifled my aspirations and passions.

Yet, it was the mental and emotional toll that cut the deepest. The vibrant colors of life dulled to a muted gray as the medication's grip tightened. My once-lively spirit waned, smothered by a numbing fog that blocked the full spectrum of human emotions. The nuances of joy, sorrow, and excitement dissipated, leaving behind a hollow shell yearning for authenticity.

The Silent Trade-Off - With each passing day, I grappled with the weighty question—did the relief the medication provided outweigh the collateral damage it exacted? Was the sacrifice of my vibrant self and the erosion of my overall well-being a fair trade-off?

The answers eluded me, buried beneath the complexities of personal experience and individual biology. It was a precarious tightrope walk, balancing the potential benefits against the mounting costs. The invisible scales of judgment teetered, never quite finding equilibrium.

Seeking Liberation - As the impact of medication gnawed at my spirit, I found solace in the stories of others who had ventured down similar paths. Their experiences echoed the dissonance I felt, validating the struggle of finding equilibrium amidst the cacophony of side effects. It was through their narratives that I glimpsed the possibility of liberation—a life beyond the captivity of medication-induced chains.

Embracing the Alternatives - In my journey to reclaim agency over my well-being, I began to explore alternative avenues. Natural therapies, mindfulness practices, and an unwavering commitment to self-care emerged as beacons of hope in a storm of uncertainty. I sought out medical professionals who understood the delicate balance between physical and mental health, and who recognized the nuanced interplay between medication and holistic well-being.

The Balance Within - As I stand on the precipice of a new chapter, I recognize that the effects of medication may erode a sense of self, but they do not define my journey. I navigate the complexities of finding equilibrium, aware that the answers may never be steadfast.

It is a dance of self-discovery, where the scales may tip in unexpected directions, questioning the purpose of medication, but also exploring the boundaries of personal agency and resilience. In this delicate balance, I continue to search for a nuanced understanding, where the true worth of medication can be assessed beyond its immediate relief, and where my own sense of self can flourish once more.

As I close this chapter of my life, marked by struggle and triumph, I reflect on how far I've come. Medication has given me the strength to face each day with renewed hope. It's not the end of my journey; rather, it's a new beginning. The threads of my mental and physical health are forever intertwined, and I embrace the knowledge that I am whole.

CHAPTER 8:

Navigating Complex Emotions: Sibling Reflections

I am his protector. I am his surrogate Mom. He is my lighthouse to remind me of service to others. He was my first recipient of impact. I am a child of God first and foremost. I am a daughter, sister, and friend. I am a social worker, and public health analyst. Public service is the nexus of all.

I sacrifice my safety and security to make sure he is okay, losing myself in a flurry of his care taking, at the playground and camp, denying myself. I wanted to protect. I knew he was different and to a great magnitude, even helping my Mom.

In the dimly lit room, shadows danced on the walls as the night wrapped its arms around my small figure nestled in bed. My eyes heavy with sleep, watched quietly as my mother's gentle embrace enveloped my brother in a cocoon of love and comfort.

As I lay there, heart heavy with a mix of emotions, I couldn't help but feel a twinge of jealousy. My brother's needs commanded attention, love, and care - qualities that often seemed to be in short supply when it came to me. I closed my eyes, trying to push away the feelings of resentment and envy that threatened to consume me. I longed for my mother's attention, the kind that was freely given to my brother.

But as I listened to the rhythmic sound of my mother's murmurs, soothing my brother into a peaceful slumber, a sense of guilt washed over me. As I sit down to write about the conundrum that has weighed heavily on my heart for so long, I find myself grappling with a whirlwind of conflicting emotions. How do you reconcile the deep love and responsibility you feel for a special needs brother with the twinges of jealousy that sometimes arise within you? It's a delicate dance, one that I have stumbled through more times than I care to admit.

Growing up with a special needs sibling can be both a blessing and a burden. You are taught the virtues of compassion, patience, and understanding from a young age, virtues that shape you into a kinder and more empathetic person. But, alongside these invaluable lessons come moments of doubt, resentment, and guilt. The feeling of jealousy can creep in unexpectedly, like an unwelcome guest at a family gathering.

It's a feeling that pricks at your conscience, whispering cruel insinuations of selfishness and inadequacy. In my experience, the key to navigating these turbulent emotions lies in acknowledging them without judgment. It's okay to feel jealous; it's a natural human emotion, not a reflection of your love for your brother. By giving yourself permission to feel and explore these emotions, you can begin to unravel the tangled knot of guilt and resentment that has taken root in your heart.

Communication is another vital tool in this journey of self-discovery. Talking openly and honestly with trusted friends or family members can provide a fresh perspective and offer much-needed support. Sometimes, simply voicing your fears and insecurities out loud can lessen their hold on you, allowing you to breathe a little easier. Above all else, it's crucial to remember that you are not alone in this struggle. Many siblings of special needs individuals grapple with similar emotions, often in silence. By sharing your story and seeking solace in the stories of others, you can find strength in community and solidarity.

As I conclude this chapter, I am reminded of the profound connection that binds siblings together, transcending differences in ability and experience. It is a bond forged in the crucible of love, tested by trials of jealousy and guilt, yet resilient in its depth and endurance. May we navigate this conundrum with grace and compassion, emerging on the other side with hearts full of understanding and acceptance.

CHAPTER 9:

PANIC – MENTAL HEALTH AND ANXIETY

It hits you hard as if you're driving at full speed into a concrete wall. Mine usually happens when I'm driving, late at night. My heart races and my breathing gets shallow. My body shakes. My eyes begin to twitch. In the moment, I have no idea what to do. I feel terrified, yet my inner strength begins to kick in. My mind clears, and I regain control.

This is a panic attack.

On my brother's 16th birthday, my Mom and I decorated the whole house.

Right before the first guests arrived, I turned to Mom and said, "Mom, I feel overwhelmed. What should I do when the kids come? What is my responsibility?"

I remember her astonishment at my questioning.

"Andrea, are you alright? You just have to..." The rest of her sentence was washed away by the cloud of confusion that slowly engulfed my shattering mind and psyche. It was a powerful feeling.

A lot is ahead of me. Right now, I have been mentally and emotionally stable for ten months. It has been a miracle, thanks to God. I am truly happy. I feel blessed. I have my priorities in order. I have goals. I have a loving and supportive family. I am being watched carefully by an amazing psychiatrist and an amazing social worker. Yes, I have been on many cocktails of psychotropic medications. I was finally put on the correct cocktail upon leaving the hospital for the second time. There are people out there who do not get medicated at all because of finances, bad providers, no support, no resources, and more. God has been good to me. I prayed to be where I am now and for Him to use me in a way that will be helpful to myself and other people.

At times, I lose hope, especially when I have panic attacks. They feel like I am dying, which is one of my present fears. I have prayed for my anxiety to go away, and it has in many ways. I have gradually met small goals. It is all about pacing oneself and not allowing yourself to be void of hope and faith. God always has a plan.

The car interior is dimly lit, with the rhythmic hum of the engine providing a soothing backdrop. I sat tensely behind the wheel, gripping it tightly as the passing headlights cast fleeting shadows across her face.

I was in my late 20s. I take deep breaths in an attempt to calm herself. However, the panic began to take hold.

(whispering to myself)

Just keep breathing… You can do this.

My heart races and my hands start to tremble uncontrollably, causing the steering wheel to shake. Beads of sweat form on my forehead, and my vision blurs slightly.

I was experiencing panic attacks while driving. I was teary-eyed Anna, clutching the steering wheel, struggling to catch my breath.

My breath quickens, and the tightness in my chest becomes more pronounced. I feel an overwhelming sense of dread wash over her.

(whispering, panicked)

I can't…I can't breathe. Please, not now.

I desperately search for a way to escape the mounting panic. My trembling hand reaches for a bottle of water in the cup holder and takes a sip. The cool liquid soothes my throat and provides a moment of relief.

Miniature streaks of light, created by approaching cars, blur into long, glowing lines against the dark backdrop. My panic has momentarily subsided, but my body is still tense, anticipating the return of anxiety.

My grip on the steering wheel tightens, my knuckles turning white. My breathing comes in short gasps, and perspiration drips down my temples.

(teary-eyed, pleading)

I need to find a safe place to pull over, just for a moment.

I scanned the roadside for an exit, determined to find a refuge from the all-consuming panic that threatens to engulf her. Suddenly, a sign for a rest area appears, guiding my hope.

My car rolls to a stop in an empty parking space. I slump forward, gripping the steering wheel to steady myself. Hot tears stream down my face as she finally succumbs to the overwhelming emotions.

I sit in her car, her body trembling, tears streaking her flushed cheeks. I reach into my bag and pulls out a small notebook, flipping it open to a page filled with coping mechanisms and grounding techniques.

(whispering, determined)

I won't let this control me. I'll find a way to overcome these panic attacks, even on the open road.

I take a deep breath, wipe away my tears, and focus on the techniques outlined in her notebook. With renewed resolve, I start the car, preparing to continue my journey, knowing that the road ahead may be challenging, but I won't let panic win.

My anxiety affected my ability to maintain healthy relationships, particularly romantic ones. Newer friendships, ones I made as an adult, were hard to maintain because of negative thinking. Do they really like me? Am I good enough? When I planned a party, did I prepare my place enough? Will they have enough to eat and drink? Relationships with men were impacted as well, especially when feelings of mistrust came up. Does he truly like me? Will he leave me when I need him most? Is our date going well? Did I prepare enough? What is he thinking? Will he judge me for my past?

Let's say I met a new guy; we spent a night together, and he showed interest. My automatic thoughts would be: I may come across as too needy. Will I look odd approaching him? I look and appear weird. Will I say something awkward that would reveal my lack of experience and nerves? Do I look ugly? Is he really as interested as he is showing? What did I do wrong? I blew it. I should have shown more interest.

According to cognitive behavioral therapy, the thinking errors that came into play were all-or-nothing thinking, disqualifying or discounting the positive, emotional reasoning, labeling, mental filter, mind-reading, overgeneralization, and should and must statements. All of this led to me being visibly anxious, nervous, and uptight. This overthinking was largely due to my generalized anxiety diagnosis.

And then there were the effects of my medication. I felt tired often, which prevented me from being social, particularly when I was feeling depressed. I gained a lot of weight too. So, that meant not being able to fit into clothes. My natural size is a size 8. Yes, due to medications, I went up to a size 16. I loved to dress up. I have been that way since the age of 11. I also enjoyed dressing up when going out. So, when I could not fit into my clothing, it was a huge blow to me. When I was small (my weight fluctuated), I felt confident and in control. When I was large, I had low self-esteem.

To my family, friends, mentors, and co-workers, to all whom I call family and friends, to my family, my many aunts and uncles, my dearest friends and confidants, my mentors, and all of you whom I call friends and family, this is for you.

One of my prayers to my Father above is for Him to help me see me the way He sees me. When I see you all, I see God's face. His bright countenance and abundant grace. His boundless love overfloweth for me. His solid support is like a tall tree. In you all, that is what I see. You are like an eagle's wings on which I soar. Where I saw in me little, you saw more. On your shoulders, I stand proud and tall. It is you who guided, supported, encouraged, adored, and believed in me when I felt small. Every victory you each, in different ways, cheered me on. There are so many wrong turns and paths I could have gone. There were times when my heart, mind, soul, and feet knew not where to turn. But God sent you angels my way so I would not crash and burn. But those of you who have know-how helped me keep my head screwed on straight. It is tempting to take shortcuts to the wrong paths. But you taught me how not to take the bait. My accomplishments are not all about me. They are mere snapshots of a long testimony. Today, I celebrate you. I celebrate love. I celebrate and sing praises to God up above because I would not be here in this place, shining in God's glory and soaking in His blessings, if it were not for you, the people I love. When I see you all, I see God's face, His bright countenance, and abundant grace. His boundless love overfloweth for me. His solid support is like a tall tree. That is what I see in you all.

My best friend, or the best of the best, is Bennett Jackson. He saw me through a whole lot. I loved him like a brother. I trust him as well, which is a difficult thing for me.

When I told him I was suffering from mental illness, he was supportive and positive. Even as I went on to tell him about the medication I took for Anxiety Disorder, he was very collected, kind, and easy-going about it. I am so glad that I have a friend like him. I need more.

I said, "The reason I have been gaining weight is because I have been taking medication. The reason I am taking medication is because

I am suffering from Anxiety Disorder and Social Phobia."

His words to me were, "This does not change what I feel about you as a friend. You are still you. Besides, I knew you were going through something. When I did not hear from you, I said to myself,

Andrea is taking care of business."

I began to cry. God was in that moment. I thank Him. Bennett is the only friend I trust enough to talk about my deepest issues. I know he will not stand in judgment of me. He will not spread my personal business to others. It is trust that led my tongue on that breezy December day. Bennett and I first met in pre-kindergarten. We lost touch when he moved to Texas in our 20s.

When I felt anxious, I was overwhelmed, tense, and frustrated. My stressors were Amaadi's behavior, group settings where I felt put on the spot, telephone conversations, and family members not being attentive to something I said.

Anxiety does not kill. Anxiety is a liar. It distorts the truth. It sends alarms through our minds and triggers our body's physical defenses. Know you will be alright. You will get through this temporary discomfort. At the same time, greet this discomfort. Do not run and hide from it. Allow yourself to feel every pulse, heartbeat, and every drop of sweat. Breathe throughout the process of facing it. I assure you, that when you do this, no matter how long it takes, the anxiety will stop. In general, anxiety is very treatable and can be overcome. Practice positive self-talk. Learn breathing and meditation techniques. Do not be ashamed to engage in talk therapy. It will be okay. Also, be around people who will see your humanity. Be around people who do not just see your flaws, but who lift you up. Be around people who will not see you as only your problems, but rather people who are in tune with your greatness as well.

CHAPTER 10:

GRAD SCHOOL – MENTAL HEALTH AND CBT

Living in New York City was a dream come true. My friends and I painted the town red. We would go out constantly, living our best lives. We went to parties, and we were free. We hopped from block to block with all the energy in the world! I graduated with a high GPA.

I was a student at Crayton University School of Social Work. I was amazed at how far I had come. I felt like a natural-born social worker. I was created to heal, as my mother says. That is my service. I healed through my words. I healed others with my poetry. I healed others with my calming presence. I was being trained at Crayton to hone my skills as a social worker and to be trained to change lives in a big way. I found myself looking around my apartment. It was surreal. I was still digesting and processing the fact that I am a student at this Ivy League School and premiere school of social work. No more tears! No more doubts!

No more fears! I am loved! I am loved by my family…I am free!

However, I still lived in a limbo between anxiety and being healed, as illustrated below.

CBT stands for Cognitive Behavioral Therapy. It is a widely recognized and evidence-based form of psychotherapy that focuses on the relationship between thoughts, emotions, and behaviors. CBT operates under the belief that our thoughts and beliefs directly influence our emotions and actions.

In CBT, a therapist works collaboratively with a person to identify and challenge negative or unhelpful thought patterns and beliefs. By doing so, individuals can learn to replace negative thoughts with more realistic and positive ones, resulting in improved emotional well-being and healthier behaviors.

CBT techniques may include various strategies such as keeping thought records, setting realistic goals, learning relaxation techniques, and engaging in behavioral experiments to test certain beliefs or assumptions. The ultimate aim of CBT is to enable individuals to develop healthier coping mechanisms, improve problem-solving skills, and cultivate more adaptive thoughts and behaviors.

CBT is commonly used to address a wide range of mental health conditions, including anxiety disorders, depression, eating disorders, addiction, and post-traumatic stress disorder (PTSD). It is typically offered in a structured and time-limited format, with regular sessions that focus on specific therapeutic goals.

It's important to note that while CBT is highly effective for many individuals, it may not be suitable for everyone. Different therapeutic approaches may be more appropriate depending on individual needs and circumstances. It is always advisable to consult with a mental health professional to determine the most suitable treatment approach.

Here were some of my journal entries at the time:

February 17th, 2011: *Class role play. I did very well and got great feedback. I wanted to do it because I felt comfortable with the material. But I was nervous. I was worried about forgetting the components of the role play. I was worried about showing my nerves and sounding nervous.*

February 18, 2011: *I do not want to be observed by my supervisor during one of my sessions.*

February 19, 2011: *I keep talking and thinking about mapping out my semester and getting on top of establishing key people for my second year internship and concentration. I have so many things to do and people to contact before the end of the year. I have to organize my assignments for the remainder of the semester. Instead, I took naps, watched TV, spent time with a friend who was online, went to a church event, and worked on further pestoni responsibilities, which have been piling up. This includes small tasks, for example, emails for inquiries about the second-year field placement process, cleaning, and packing for the weekend. I also feel like I have to put other things on hold until I take the first step and complete an urgent task, for example, process recordings. I didn't go to the gym or pack for my weekend on time, for example.*

February 19th, 2011, continued: *I have been procrastinating in a big way with my process recordings. I do not do them right away. My supervisor has pointed out that it is an inconvenience a few times. Instead of completing them on Friday, I waited until Saturday afternoon. My supervisor does not want to receive them after 7:00 PM on Saturdays. I feel stressed about having to do them because it takes time, and I'm self-conscious about my memory, which is counterintuitive because completing them right after my sessions would make more sense.*

February 20th, 2011: *I had a great time spending time with family and friends in Connecticut. I had no worries. I was off from work on Monday and Tuesday.*

February 22nd, 2011: *Worry set in because I had not started my work for the week and had not planned for the next two busy months. I felt preoccupied with worrisome thoughts. "Can I do it?" I felt overwhelmed. I felt stuck. "Where to begin?" Major decisions within the next two weeks. Major assignments are due in the next two months back to back. Self-deprecating.*

February 22nd, 2011, continued: *An argument with mom. She did something that was out of line. In the midst of the argument, I became enraged. I don't normally go into fits of rage, so it scared me. I threw my phone three times. I was palpitating slightly. Shallow breathing. Somewhat panicky. I went into my room to calm down—cried, prayed, breathed. I was able to clearly and calmly articulate my frustration to my mom later that night and the next morning. She apologized.*

February 23rd, 2011: *No work done, no plan made. Feeling anxious and overwhelmed. I have to leave for school in an hour. Now in damage control mode completing the reading assignment that is due for the day. Feel unproductive wondering, "When will I get organized?" "Why am I giving myself stress?"*

February 23rd, 2011, continued: *I submitted a paper one hour and 45 minutes late. Beforehand, I pushed it off. The thought of racing to finish the assignment by the midnight deadline caused me a lot of anxiety. Worry set in. As I was worried about completing the assignment, my long list of other responsibilities flooded my mind. I was particularly distressed at the news, and my top choice for a few placements for my second year is not an option for me. I became emotional when I heard the news. I talked it over with a friend and my mom.*

February 24th, 2011: *I noticed that during a class discussion, I felt self-conscious and anxious. I was self-conscious of being stared at and looking nervous because when I feel bouts of anxiety, nervousness accompanies it. I felt anxiety physically with tension in my stomach, throat, chest, and forehead. It felt odd. This sometimes happens when I feel put on the spot.*

On February 25th, 2011: *I attended a Crayton school social work mixer. I met a great guy, Danny. He is perfect for me. He's very handsome, tall, and smart, and we share the same background—exactly my type. We chatted briefly at first. He introduced himself. I left his side to mingle with other people. He began speaking to a friend of mine who told him I was from Ghana. He got excited. We began to talk at length. I felt comfortable during our first conversation. We kicked it off.*

Once I realized that I was attracted, I began to get nervous. When I started getting nervous, I began to feel self-conscious. The third time, we spoke alone at the bar in the lounge. I wanted to exchange information, but I felt too shy to bring it up, although we got along really well, and he appeared very interested.

I left his side for a third time to talk to friends. Express that I was interested in him to them. But I told him I was too shy to get his number. They were surprised. I felt nervous about approaching him again. I didn't even want to let on that I liked him. Whenever my friends would start talking about him, and I felt he could overhear, I told them to quiet down. They were amused but also surprised. I question whether I should approach him and ask for his number. I didn't want to appear aggressive. There were a few opportunities for me to engage in conversation with him again. I did not take them. This went on for a while. I gathered the courage to approach him again only because a group of friends was standing close by.

I did have courage, though, and approached him a couple of times at the beginning of the night, even when friends were not around. The thoughts that went through my mind in between contact with him were, Will I look awkward approaching him at this time? Will it be obvious that I like him? Will I say something awkward that would hint at my lack of experience? My face recently broke out, so do I look bad tonight?

Finally, we spoke again. I felt comfortable approaching him because he was around a friend of mine. We began to talk again. He invited me to a party his friend was having at a club. I said, "Maybe, it depends on what my friends want to do." In my mind, I wanted to exchange information. Thankfully, during our interaction, he brought up that he did not give me the information about his friend's party.

So, at that point, we exchanged information. I felt relieved because I thought I had lost my chance. When it came time for my friends and me to go to another bar, I felt shy to say goodbye. He spoke with two other people. I gathered courage and went up to him and said it was great meeting him. I wanted to say more. But I ended up shaking his hand, which felt awkward. We left my friends. As we made our way to the next bar, he called me. He asked if my friends and I would like to go to his friend's party. He said he called because he was leaving the bar and was driving and thought we would want to drive with him instead of taking the subway. I thought, how nice. He is showing interest again. I said no because I told him the entire group was split up, and I was unsure who wanted to go. I rambled an answer, though I was flattered and hoped to stay in touch. I thought this was a good sign, a sign that he liked me.

He left for his friend's party. We all went to the bar. After a considerable amount of time, I asked my friend if she would have liked to go to the party. She said she was interested. At one point, she said she was somewhat tired. I begged her to go. I did not want to be alone with him. I was also interested, unhappy at the prospect of seeing him again. I called him. He was a long way away, headed to the party. We waited for about 35 minutes or more. He came back to the area to pick us up. When he first said alright, I was thrilled. This was a sign that he liked me and wanted to hang out, especially since he was almost at the party when he turned around. I felt great. I sat in the front with him. I felt nervous to talk. I did not want to say anything stupid or awkward. I also did not want to sound as nervous as I was. I questioned whether or not he liked me, though he showed a lot of interest in the conversation and action.

At the party, he grabbed me onto the dance floor. We danced for a while. He danced in an intimate "I'm interested and attracted to you" way. The DJ made a comment, pointing us out on the dance floor. He said something to the effect of, "I should get his information." The chemistry was very much there. At one point, the DJ said, "Grab a single lady." Danny says something to the effect that he found someone referring to me. I made a flirty comment that he was lucky he already had one.

We went to another floor of the club. That is when everything changed. We danced on and off. The chemistry was still there each time. I still felt nervous in between interactions when I would want to approach him again. At one point, he met another girl at the club. My heart sank. I began to question myself. What did I do wrong? Did I come off nervous?

How do I approach him now? I even felt nervous around his friends. I thought to myself, He's probably already talked to them about me. I feel awkward with the other girl now in the picture. Are they judging me? Is he comparing the two of us? Do I look alright? Is it my weight? I felt so defeated.

He would still come to find me on the dance floor. The chemistry was still there, but he was also interacting with the other girl, dancing and talking. At one point, we locked eyes on the dance floor while he was dancing with the other girl. I quickly looked away. I thought to myself, I blew it. For the rest of the night, I remained cool and collected, though I was dying inside to have his complete attention again. By the end of the night, I felt I had lost the battle. It appeared that he was kicking it off with the other girl. She even came to the VIP section where we were all at, and they talked. I gave up and accepted defeat. I thought to myself, I should have been more confident and shown more interest. I felt self-conscious at the end of the night whenever I would go over to our section. I felt his friends were looking at me and judging me and that they felt the other girl was better for him and more attractive.

One of his best friends called me over to dance. I hesitated. I thought to myself, Is he doing this out of pity? Do I look pathetic? When he escorted me and my friends out as we left, I thought to myself, I am in the friend zone now. I lost his interest. I should have flirted more. He thinks I am weird.

I am hopeful that I will have more opportunities since he works and goes to my school. I just hope that I can express my true feelings. On the car ride home, my friend asked me, "Why are you so shy?" I said, "With guys?" She said, "Yes, you don't have to be. Why do you do that?" She makes comments along the lines that I don't need to be. I am beautiful. Be a little more aggressive and flirty. She was confused by my behavior. I said, "You wouldn't think that I am like that with guys, would you?" She said, "No." I thought to myself, She is right. I have to fix this behavior. Otherwise, I'll remain single, and guys like Danny will slip through my fingers always.

February 25th, 2011, continued: *In addition to this situation with Danny, I experienced other bouts of anxiety in the environment I was in. When I had the conversion disorder, there was an agoraphobic component to it too. When I was at a party with* *fluorescent lights flashing, it would trigger my conversion symptoms—the rolling of the eyes. I find that though I do not have conversion disorder anymore, I experience anxiety with the same trigger. When I was at the lounge in the club afterward, the lights bothered me. I worry that it will trigger panic within me. I worried that I would experience dissociation. In my mind, I mapped out where I would exit if I began to have symptoms of a panic attack. While these thoughts went through my mind, I felt my heart racing. At times, I would close my eyes when the club lights would flash, thinking that would calm me down. I stood on the side of the dancefloor a few times because I did not want to have a panic attack. My mind reverted back to years ago when my conversion symptoms were triggered by being overstimulated in my environment. I felt warm. The thoughts I mentioned above raced through my mind a few times throughout the night as soon as I stepped into this particular room of the club and noticed that there were strobing lights. That would be on the whole night the abovementioned thoughts raced through my mind, and my heart raced.*

February 26, 2011, *my mom gave me great advice about Danny. I called him, and we talked for almost an hour. I felt comfortable. I decided that I did nothing wrong last night. That was my first time meeting him. We kicked it off. He showed interest. I did more than I would normally feel comfortable doing. I am proud of myself. I have perspective, and a good friend, which is a great starting point even if things don't work out.*

February 28th, 2011: *I am worried about all of the schoolwork I have to do. I am preoccupied with all of the internship stuff I have to do. I did make essential appointments with individuals from school to prepare for my next steps. I am experiencing anxiety, anticipating my return to my field placement, and facing the new responsibilities I have group work. I am concerned about the volume of work in addition to my responsibilities at school. I am experiencing anticipatory anxiety about a presentation I have on Wednesday. I am not prepared. I have the support of family and friends.*

March 2nd, 2011: *Class presentation. Beforehand, I thought I had prepared that morning. Will I run out of time? Will my voice shake? Will they like it is my work? Add a quit because it was last minute. Am I going to look like I'm reading the PowerPoint the entire time, or will I sound natural? It looked good. During the presentation, the professor said, "You are the most prepared student thus far." The other presenter said, "Your PowerPoint looks better than mine." I felt the tension in my throat and stomach, but it was very low compared to what I thought I would feel. I felt comfortable. Only worried about going overtime.*

Afterward, I thought I felt I did a great job. The audience appeared to like it. I read one of the feedback notes. April was a lot of information, and a con was reading off of the slides. By chance, I spoke with the girl who wrote that feedback. I told her I created the presentation this morning and didn't have time to memorize the slides. She was impressed. Then it was, "Oh no! I may have emphasized the wrong points." But, all the feedback I received on my presentation was positive. I also received a good grade.

March 3rd, 2011: *I was anxious, overwhelmed, and pessimistic about my meeting with the director of DC field placements. Before I walked in the door, I was not sure what to expect. I wanted an internship in DC so badly. I expected possible rejection or difficulty convincing her. A minute into the meeting, their director assured me of a DC internship. I went in there knowing exactly what I wanted. I conveyed that and got the internship. Not only that, but I do not have to go through the selection process like everyone else. My placement for next year is set. That evening, I had a meeting with my advisor, I was excited about my second-year field placement. Based on history, I thought that my advisor would be unsupportive. Rather, she was extremely helpful. During the meeting, by chance and what I call a miracle, an alumnus of my school approached us because he overheard our conversation. He was in the same concentration as I was. He had a field placement in DC. He* *also had a fellowship that I will be applying for next academic year. Since our meeting, he has given me contacts and advice on DC field placements, specific agencies, and our concentration. I felt so encouraged after the meeting.*

On March 18th, 2011, Friday night: *I attended a mixer for students of color from my program. It was held at a lounge in the village. A guy that I'm interested in, Danny, was there with his friends. Our interaction was fine. I was myself most of the night. At the end of the night, Danny and his friends wanted to hang out further with friends and me from school. As we were approaching the next location, I noticed that I was experiencing anxiety. My central thoughts were, Will I experience dissociation? Will my anxiety be triggered by the cramped, smoky hookah bar? Throughout the rest of the night, I experienced this anxiety book before we arrived there and for the duration of us hanging out at the bar. At one point, we decided we were going to a club. Though this was something I wanted to do, I felt more anxious.*

April 7th, 2011: *I felt quite self-conscious during my direct practice class. This sometimes happens when I am in class. Though I like to speak up and participate, often, I felt awkward and anxious when attention was drawn in my direction, whether it was someone next to me speaking or any other attention paid in my physical direction. My feelings and thoughts were jittery, I am being stared at, I feel twitchy as a result, do I look nervous, how strange, heart beating, conscious of my movements and facial expressions. I felt worried about the poor grade I received in my advocacy class. I wondered if I could recover from the grade. My goal is to get into the class. I have two major projects due by the end of the semester to redeem and bring up my average. I took a leadership role in my group project, which is worth a lot. I secured great contacts and created an entire plan to ensure a great grade for our final project, which is worth a lot. I decided* *not to look backward in fear but to keep moving forward on the next project. I attribute this attitude to our talks about catastrophizing and my faith in God.*

April 7th, 2011 continued: *I participated in a school-sponsored event in which I performed my poetry. Before getting there, I felt nervous.*

The thoughts and emotions were, will I sound nervous? I read I don't memorize my poetry, so will I look foolish? Will I deliver well? In the moments leading up to my turn to perform, I felt anxious. I felt it in my stomach and throat. When my friends and others were speaking to me, all I could think of was my anxiety over my performance. I was also preoccupied with the fact that the venue did not have a mic stand, and I was planning on reading from a journal. I thought I would look awkward holding the mic and flipping the page. While I was performing, I could tell that I appeared and sounded nervous. I worried that people would notice my nerves. I recalled comments about people who could not read my mind or see my emotions. That helped. After my performance, people approached me and said they liked my poems. I was still fixated on my nerves showing. So, I asked other performers how they thought I did. Their feedback was positive. But I was not convinced. I did focus, however, on one girl who said, "It must be hard to get up there and perform. Do you always read, or do you memorize too?"

April 7th, 2011, continued: *I focused on what I perceived to be the negative feedback that fed into my insecurities.*

April 8th, 2011, late Thursday night: *The guy I'm interested in contacting me. I have been excited lately that he continues to show genuine interest in getting to know me. Though I feel frustrated that things have not progressed towards dating, I feel that this is a good starting point. We talked for some time that night. I felt positive and good about our interaction. We connected very well. At one point in the conversation, he commented, in a good way, about* *how I am always smiling. But then my optimism turned into doubt. He said something that puzzled me at first, then discouraged me later. My smile reminded him of innocent happiness. I began to try to understand what he said. I asked and told him I thought he meant like happy, open, and innocent. Then he said in response, "I was thinking along the lines of not being exposed to the elements and harshness of life, a child, a baby." I thought to myself, here we go again, a guy noticing my lack of experience with relationships. I jumped to the conclusion that I am sure he was not likely thinking. He said he was responding to my interpretation of the phrase. The phrase only applied to my smile. At the end of the conversation, he said I guess I'll see you around. I once again focused on the negative and said to myself, I am in the friend zone. I completely ignored the fact that we had a great conversation and connected the fact we spoke for a while. We even wrote a poem together entitled "Innocent Happiness." We made light of the phrase. But still, I felt negative. I invited him to a dinner party I hosted on Saturday night. He came with his sister. I thought this was a nice gesture and another sign that he wanted to get to know me. My resolve is to select go and go with the flow when it comes to him and guys in general.*

April 8th, 2011: *I sat down to plan out my schedule for the next three weeks of school. I felt overwhelmed and anxious. My thoughts and feelings were, can I do all of this? Will I be able to complete these assignments well, given that I am starting some of my finals late? Will my schedule work? I have resolved to finish off my year strong academically. To do this, I have promised myself that I would get organized. Being orderly makes me feel less anxious and in control. I did not finish my schedule. I also did not finish all the work I wanted to get done on Friday and Saturday. I began to panic about how I was going to function for the rest of the academic year. I decided to rely on faith and hard work to do my part and let God do the rest.*

April 9th, 2011: *I got a call from a guy I met a little while ago. He shared that he was interested in me, and he asked me out on a date. At one point, he said he had a question for me about my* *relationships with guys. I thought to myself, here we go again, another guy who notices my lack of experience. In examining myself and seeking counsel from friends, I have concluded that I must be at peace with who I am. I must be confident that I have a lot to offer and relationships. My past is a gift, a gift that the right guy will appreciate.*

April 9th, 2011, Saturday night: *I had a dinner party. It was great! My friends and I had a blast. The theme was a cultural potluck. Everyone brought a dish that represented their culture. It ended well. But my anxiety before the party was high. Beforehand, I worried that there would be too many people because of the number of people that my friend and I invited, the fact it was posted on Facebook as a public event, and over 60 people were on the waiting list. I was worried that I did not have enough space, that there would be too much noise in my apartment, disturbing neighbors, and that my furniture would be messed up as a result of the large numbers.*

Will I get everything ready in time? I made a conscious decision to let go, have fun, and not worry. This is a dinner I have wanted to have for a while now, and now it is happening. Everything worked out. I had a lot of help with the setup. A majority of the friends I wanted to be there were there. I was happy that my friends who did not know each other beforehand met each other. Everyone had fun. The right number of people were there.

As I resolved not to worry, I relaxed before entering the party. I prayed about it beforehand, and it all worked out. It was a success. On top of that, all the guys I was interested in came with his sister. I was ecstatic about that.

April 10th, 2011: *He called me late Sunday night. The question he wanted to know was, "When was my last relationship?" I dodged the question. I told him that I don't feel it necessary to divulge personal information until I know someone. I also told him that I feel I have been misleading and want to maintain our relationship on a friendship basis. I told him that I think he's a great guy and a lot of fun. And we would be great friends. In all honesty, I want to get to* *know him more on that level. He responded by saying that it was cool. He appreciates what I tell him. He also said he does not like to go fast when it comes to relationships with friends first. He jokingly said that I might change my mind after spending time with him. We're going out next weekend.*

April 11th, 2011: *I began to feel discouraged when I thought about all the work I had to do and had not done yet.*

April 12th, 2011: *Today, I ran another session of my bereavement group. Beforehand, I experienced anxiety from the morning. The thoughts that went through my mind were, I am the sole facilitator of this group, will I be able to remember everything that I have planned for the students for the session, and will I remember all the details of the session and write an accurate process recording? I was fortunate today because I ran into one of the guidance counselors at the school, who happens to have expertise in grief counseling. She offered to go over the plans I had for each session. She also offered to sit in to evaluate the students. She gave great tips for helping the students. Right before this session, I went over my plan for the students and gathered the materials they needed. I made a conscious decision to put my worries and insecurities about my memory and performance aside and focus on the students and their well-being. So far, they appear to be getting a lot out of the group. The first session went well. They were very supportive of one another. They were engaged and participated. They were comfortable, which was evident since they divulged a lot of personal information early on. It has been an excellent group so far.*

April 12, 2011, continued: *As a sole facilitator of a group with no prior experience running groups, I am proud that I have done well. I have been able to be creative in control and help students through their grieving process by providing a safe space for them to unload their emotions. It is a rewarding experience to be able to help them and to see them progress. This second session went well in terms of the student's progress. They shared even more today. They were very comfortable and verbalized that they felt lighter after the session.*

When I did a one-word check-in with them at the end, one student said he felt "free," and the other students said happily, "This was an improvement on their end." Throughout the session, I was nervous. It did not show, but in my mind, I could not help but worry about how I was going to remember all of the details. I feel that taking notes breaks up the flow of a session. I am practicing writing notes after each session. I have been successful thus far. I have run four group sessions so far, and for each one, I have been able to write detailed process recordings afterward. I am proud of that and the fact that I am running two groups without a problem. Running two groups and writing process recordings for each of them was something I dreaded beforehand. Now I realize that I am more than capable, as evidenced by the outcome of these sessions. I have conquered a fear and faced my anxiety heading on. Group work and my insecurity about my memory were two of my major goals before starting at CUCARD. I am proud of myself.

I can say the same for other goals I have set. Even though she was there to observe the students, I felt slightly nervous about the guidance counselor sitting in on the session. I thought to myself, What if I do poorly in front of her? After the session, I asked her if she would be willing to help me with my process recording. She said she did not mind going over the session with me. She added, "You have nothing to worry about. You did a great job." She also said my supervisor likes me a lot. She added that she would put in a good word for me to my supervisor.

Even though it was tough, I did it. Though I battled with anxiety heavily, I was still able to accomplish a lot. Trials are not meant to hold you down. Some people are built to endure. God gives his toughest battles to His strongest soldiers.

CHAPTER 11:

MENTAL ILLNESS – MENTAL HEALTH AND STIGMA

Mental illness does not define who you are. You are more than your illness. I am a writer. I am a social worker. I am a public health professional. Mental illness did not change any of this. I just have something new to write and speak about. As I reflect on the past, I realize I am not my imperfections nor my flaws, nor my negative experiences. In fact, my imperfections and flaws add to my experiences. They have helped me to bless the lives of others. I have accomplished so much in my life. If it had not been for my pitfalls, I would not have been able to do either. I am not a victim. I am a victor. I am powerful beyond measure.

In the future, I hope to meet my forever person who will accept me for who I am. I anticipate starting a family of my own. Aside from someone who's attractive and kind, I want someone who will be understanding and supportive of my mental health history. I also want someone who is understanding, supportive, and kind about my brother Amaadi's condition. I want someone who is culturally aware.

I want someone who is respectful and interested in my culture. I want someone who is God-fearing and Christian. I want someone intelligent. And I want someone who is smart about finances. Journal entry:

August 22, 2018: My Partner Wishlist

1.   **Personality:** funny/sense of humor; affectionate (I lack this.); kind (doesn't put others down)

2.   **Qualities:** learned, smart, ambitious with action; adventurous (loves to try new things and have new experiences in the world, i.e., traveling); mature; actively fulfilling their divine PURPOSE in life (not just degrees, but actively working towards goals)

3.   **Physical attributes:** tall; any race; attractive

4.   **Character:** strong morals; Christian; and playful

5.   **Deal breakers:** lazy (not fulfilling divine purpose); no sense of humor; dishonest

I offer all of these things. I have been in love twice. The first time, things ended because I was more mature and further along in life than the person was. The second time, the person had a lot of baggage. And, we never fully shared our stories. I thank God every day for all of my experiences, both good and bad. The good experiences were fun. The bad experiences built character and strength and made me a living testimony. I want to give back to my community, my country, and to those who I don't know whose stories are just like mine. I want to help them get through the hard moments. I know that not everybody needs to know my story. However, I believe it is very important for everyone to share their stories. We do not go through things for ourselves. We did not suffer because God was punishing us.

Rather, we go through things and suffer to be a blueprint of survival for those with similar struggles. It is selfish to keep our stories to ourselves. We have a responsibility to share our testimonies. There are lives on the brink of ending that can be saved by telling our stories. I am more than what was meant for my demise. There was a plan for my defeat, but I never gave up. The enemy will never have a foothold on me. My backbone is erect and stable as a tree. I have no more tears. I have no more fears. I have no more guilt. I have no more shame.

My heavenly Father is ever-present and near. Never will he leave me to fight on my own. My history has consistently shown. Never will I fall too hard to rise up. Never will the enemy shut this girl up. Faith and hope and promises anew. His will be done. I have already won. I write this through tears because it has been hard. There were many scary moments. Before I knew my purpose, I asked God why. I did not understand why I was being punished. It did not make sense to me. Little did I know, He was by my side throughout it all. When I discovered who He was, I learned that there was a purpose for my life. I did not suffer in vain. I have touched tens and thousands of lives. I fight for my family. And I fight for those tens and thousands whom I do not know. The enemy lied to me, making me feel like I was all alone.

God sends angels our way to help us. We must use the pain we go through as healing for ourselves and the healing of others. You are more than your illness. God never leaves you. I still have hope that all will be well and that my happy ending is on its way.

Mental illness is not a death sentence. The stigma surrounding mental illness should not defeat a person. Life goes on after a diagnosis.

It is possible to lead a normal life, and it is possible to be a functional person despite one's illness.

A Whisper in the Shadows -

In the depths of my mind, a whisper began to grow louder. At first, I dismissed it as just a passing thought, but soon it transformed into an all-consuming presence. The weight of invisible chains bound me, keeping my voice stifled and my pain hidden. This was the beginning of my journey through the twisted landscape of mental illness and the stigma that encased it.

Lost in the Labyrinth -

Navigating my way through the labyrinthine maze of mental illness was a daunting task. Each step felt heavy with judgment, every confession laced with fear. The stigma that clung to mental health issues was like a suffocating fog, casting doubt on the validity of my struggles and isolating me from those who might understand.

Masks and Masquerades -

To survive in a world that stigmatized mental health, I learned to wear masks. Smiling faces hid crumbling souls, laughter echoing through hollow hearts. I became skilled at pretending, expertly concealing the invisible battles raging within. But behind closed doors, the masks grew heavy, and the burden of secrecy weighed me down.

Breaking the Silence -

One day, I found solace in the words of others who had dared to break the silence. Their stories echoed through my veins, igniting a fire within me. It was time to shatter the chains of stigma and share my truth with the world. My voice, once muted, grew stronger with every word spoken, every vulnerable admission uttered.

Unveiling the Monsters -

As I bravely revealed my mental health struggles, I faced a wall of judgment and misunderstanding. Ignorance fueled the fires of prejudice, while myths and misconceptions held tight to societal beliefs. The monsters of stigma loomed large, threatening to consume me. But I refused to be silenced.

The Power of Understanding -

In the face of stigma, I sought understanding. I reached out to friends, family, and even strangers, aiming to educate and destigmatize mental health. Through conversations, I dispelled myths, shared personal experiences, and shed light on the realities of living with a mental illness. Each connection formed a thread in a tapestry of empathy and compassion.

The Strength in Vulnerability -

I discovered strength in vulnerability, embracing every scar and every tear as a testament to my resilience. By openly sharing my story, I empowered others to do the same. Together, we shattered the illusion of weakness and embraced the power of acceptance and support.

Towards Wholeness -

Through my journey, I realized that mental health is not separate from our overall well-being but an integral part of our wholeness. I learned to prioritize self-care, seek therapy, and embrace the support of loved ones. In doing so, I blazed a trail towards a more compassionate and understanding society.

A New Beginning -

As I close this chapter of my life, I understand that the battle against mental health stigma is ongoing. But I am no longer held captive by its chains. I walk forward with a renewed purpose, advocating for change, and fighting for a world where mental health is embraced, stigma is shattered, and wholeness is celebrated.

CONCLUSION

Pain is your biggest asset. There is always a purpose to it.

And, we can always use our pain to help others. We do this by sharing our pain. In fact, sharing our pain is the blueprint to healing. Telling your story helps you heal. And, it helps others. We do not go through things for ourselves. We do not go through things in vain. There is always a purpose to pain. Expressing your pain can be of huge help to other people going through similar things. In fact, connecting with others is *part* of the healing process.

If you are going through mental illness, believe me— there are other people you know who are experiencing something similar. Someone has to be brave enough to trust, to believe that telling your story, even the ugly parts, will connect you with those around you and be a blueprint, a pathway, for your own healing. No matter where you are on the journey of mental illness—your story has the potential to save you.

I am grateful for all of my experiences, both good and bad. The good experiences were fun. The bad experiences built character and strength in me.

I want to give back to my community, my country, and to those who I don't know whose stories are just like mine. I want to help them get through the hard moments. I know that not everybody needs to know my story, but I've written it as a memoir. They told me to Journal, to help those who do.

Consider what stories YOU need to share with someone in your life—the ugly kind, the unfinished story, the messy middle.

Recovery from mental illness is a journey, and by sharing our stories, we are able to get the support we need as well as inspire others in their own recovery.

We reduce stigma by sharing our stories, whether we have a mental illness or are having a bad day. And, when we do that, everyone gets to tell their story and use their pain to both heal themselves and heal others.

Pain truly is your biggest asset. You may not have discovered that in your own life yet. When you do, it has the potential to transform your emotional well-being. When I look back at the year I took off school, it felt horrible at that time, but I would not change it for the world. Because that pain I went through helped me heal and is now helping others heal.

Whether you yourself are experiencing mental illness, you know someone who is, or you're just in the middle of a difficult place—perhaps a financial crisis, loss of a loved one, or any other tragedy—we ALL can benefit from telling our stories. How do we create an environment where everyone can tell their story freely, without judgment or stigma? How can we practice telling our painful stories?

Your life is a blueprint for somebody else's survival. I want you to believe as I do that we go through challenges in order to help other people. That pain can be our greatest asset, if we share it. The great Maya Angelou said: "There is no greater agony than being an untold story inside you." And I encourage you to tell yours. I thank God every day for all of my experiences, both good and bad. The good experiences were fun. The bad experiences built character and strength and made me a living testimony. I want to give back to my community, my country, and to those who I don't know whose stories are just like mine. I want to help them get through the hard moments. I know that not everybody needs to know my story. However, I believe it is very important for everyone to share their stories. We do not go through things for ourselves. We did not suffer because God was punishing us.

My heavenly Father is ever-present and near. Never will he leave me to fight on my own. My history has consistently shown. Never will I fall too hard to rise up. Never will the enemy shut this girl up. Faith and hope and promises anew. His will be done. I have already won. I write this through tears because it has been hard. There were many scary moments. Before I knew my purpose, I asked God why. I did not understand why I was being punished. It did not make sense to me. Little did I know, He was by my side throughout it all. When I discovered who He was, I learned that there was a purpose for my life.

I did not suffer in vain. I have touched tens and thousands of lives. I fight for my family. And I fight for those tens and thousands whom I do not know. The enemy lied to me, making me feel like I was all alone.

God sends angels our way to help us. We must use the pain we go through as healing for ourselves and the healing of others. You are more than your illness. God never leaves you. I still have hope that all will be well and that my happy ending is on its way.

Make It To Shore

I can't figure out what sort of tears these are.

Rivers are flooding down my cheeks.

I need to make it to dry land.

Cascade waterfalls create a beautiful landscape, masking ugly, dripping, rusty pipes.

Whitewater rapids rush, turning into quiet streams.

They are tears of a heart that has endured too much.

I let go like breaking waves on an ocean line.

I surrender all as I make it to shore into my Father's arms.

Stillness and quiet.

Peace and tranquility.

The presence of God.

I Let Go

I let go of my fears.
I let go of my worries. I let go of my anxiety.

I let go of my inhibitions. I let God take control.

I let go of my weaknesses. I

let   go   of

     my

hesitations. I let go
of the scary drive. I
let go of my fear to
die.

     I let God take control.

     I let go of my headaches.
     I let go of my
ailing psyche. I let

     go   of

     the

negativity.

     I let God take control.
     I trusted that He would
guide my path. I trusted He would
be my light.

     I trusted He would
steer my course. I trusted He
loved me a lot.
I let God take control and finally let go.

My call to action for you has seven steps:

1. **Recognition.** My recovery from mental illness has been a journey. It was a long road, but I did it. I am now at a place where I am comfortable with who I am. I owe my recovery to God, my loving and supportive family, loyal friends, skilled medical providers, a clear diagnosis, and appropriate and effective medication.

2. **Acceptance.** Accept the exterior judgment. It took me a long time to accept my diagnosis. I was ashamed for a long time, to the point where I recoiled away from close friends, keeping my experience a secret because I feared rejection. I also found myself not fully accepting that there was something wrong with me. I ultimately realized that I had true friends when they continued to accept me for who I was. I have found that the more I accept what has happened to me, the more healing gets done. This acceptance made it easier for me to disclose my struggles with mental illness to friends. It is impossible to fight mental illness on one's own. There were times when I felt that there was no need to disclose all of my concerns to health providers and family members. I felt ashamed, and I feared being labeled crazy. It is so important to be open to other people about critical mental health concerns, especially people who are there to help you.

3. **Support system.** Have trusted family and friends that you can depend on.

4. **Seek treatment.** Seek out the proper health providers for specific mental health conditions.

5. **Share your stories.** Your life is a blueprint for somebody else's survival. We go through challenges in order to help other people. We do not go through things for ourselves. We don't suffer because God is punishing us. Rather, we go through things and suffer to be a blueprint of survival for those going through similar struggles.

6. **Creative Outlets.** Sharing in different creative capacities, like poetry, art, and music, is wonderful for healing. I am a very creative person. Since the age of 10, I have expressed myself through verse. I love writing poetry. My imagination and my dreams have always been as immense and endless as the sky up

above. I love to dream. My dreams are expressed through my creative writing. Music is another passion of mine. I listen to everything: gospel, R&B, reggae, Latin, African, and rock. I sing in a band at my church. Singing has been a passion of mine since high school. I also love to dance, and I do it every chance that I get.

7. **Faith.** I am a child of God first and foremost. God is the first and the last being I speak to every day. I would not be here if it were not for Him. My parents exposed my siblings and me to faith. However, God became real to me on a personal level at a very early age. I have always been a prayerful person. However, it was not until the age of 18 that I fully devoted my life to God. I am truly in touch with my emotions, and I feel very deeply. I am sensitive. I empathize with the downtrodden and destitute. I have always been that way.

I Have Won

Am I worthy of such a degree?
Could it be possible that it is not
for me? Glory and Honor and Praise to
Thee, for bringing me far and making me
free. Guilt, shame, and fear, grip me so
tight, though I
know You're near. Hopes so high, up the
ladder I still rise.

Basking in the land of
milk and honey, in a place of
abundance, to my surprise.
Drops of tears, shouts of
joy.

A dichotomy of emotions, I cannot
control.

Honor You. I wish to do, yet, a blockage, like a clogged valve,
makes me feel like this wish
can't reach You. The clog and barricade, a deadly
creation
of my own, serves no one good, my
history has shown. So, right now I decree, as that stumbling block attempts to
return.

I am worthy of everything You have placed in me.
I am worthy of this land, flowing with things so sweet. I am worthy
of Your love and Your adoration for me.

No more fears, shame, guilt, no more tears, for my Heavenly Father
is ever present and near. Never will He leave me to fight on my own,
my history has
consistently shown. Never will I fall too hard to rise
up. Never will the Enemy shut this girl
up. I will forever honor God up
above, for His goodness, mercy
and love. Onward I go, with an
abundance of cheer. Stronger and
wiser I become every year. Never will
I look back to those dark days.

Never again will I allow myself to
reenter that place. I am a new creation. I am
like a spring flower in full bloom. In this
heart, sorrow has no room.

The enemy will never have a
foothold on me. This girl's backbone is erect
and stable like a tree. Faith and hope and

promises anew, I have been restored. God's
will be done.

   I have already won.

RESOURCES

Recommended by SAMHSA

- **988 Suicide & Crisis Lifeline**
  https://www.suicidepreventionlifeline.org/
  24-hour, toll-free, confidential suicide prevention hotline
  available to anyone in suicidal crisis or emotional distress.

- **SAMHSA's National Helpline: 1-800-662-HELP (4357)**
  https://www.samhsa.gov/find-help/national-helpline
  SAMHSA's National Helpline is a free, confidential, 24/7,
  365-day-a-year treatment referral and information service (in
  English and Spanish) for individuals and families facing
  mental and/or substance use disorders.

- **Find Treatment**
  https://findtreatment.samhsa.gov/

Online Mental Health Resources

- **Shatterproof**
  A national nonprofit with online addiction education &
  support.

- **Health Unlocked**
  A health-focused social network with communities for
  anxiety, depression, and other mental health issues.

- **Turn2Me**

Online support group for anxiety, depression, stress, and general mental health run by qualified professionals. Sessions are free but require a reservation in advance.

- **Daily Strength**
  Peer-based online forum and support group for anxiety.

- **Mental Health Forum**
  Peer-A peer-to-peer community for a range of mental health issues, from anxiety to eating disorders.

- **7 Cups**
  Free 24/7 chat with volunteer listeners. Monthly online counseling is available with a licensed therapist for a fee.

- **Bliss**
  A free, self-guided interactive therapy program for depression.

- **Mental Health America**
  A community-based nonprofit with interactive tools to get help for mental illness.

- **MentalHealth.gov**
  A comprehensive, government-sponsored guide with resources for multiple mental health issues.

Financial Hardship Resources

- **211**
  Need help right now? In many communities, dialing 2-1-1 will connect you with resources to secure basic needs, from food to housing assistance.

- **Government Benefits**

Find all available government assistance for which you may qualify.

- **Net Wish**
  Request financial assistance for particular needs up to $200.

- **Need Help Paying Bills**
  A reference for state benefit programs, rent assistance, debt relief, and money management.

- **NeedyMeds**
  A nonprofit organization that helps people find assistance to afford their medication.

- **Smart About Money**
  Free online courses for saving, health care costs, retirement, and more.

Crisis Resources

- **ReachOut**
  Mobile app offering discussions, recommendations, and support from like-minded people and a stigma-free environment.

- **The National Suicide Prevention Lifeline**
  Free 24/7 crisis support

- **The Trevor Project**
  Crisis intervention for the LGBTQ+ community

- **IMAlive**
  Online crisis network with support from trained, certified volunteers.

Mindfulness Resources

- **<u>Insight Timer</u>**
  Free app for sleep, anxiety, and stress.

- **<u>Calm</u>**
  Wellness app for better sleep, meditation, and relaxation.

- **<u>Simple Habit</u>**
  Meditation app to stress less and do more.

- **<u>Breethe</u>**
  Meditation music and personalized wellness recommendations.

- **<u>Guided Mind</u>**
  Free meditation and sleep app.

Exercise Resources

- **<u>Healthy Runners' Community</u>**
  Community and forum dedicated to mindful living through mindful running.

- **<u>Fitness Blender</u>**
  Free in-home workout videos.

- **<u>BodyFit by Amy</u>**
  Free body-positive workouts for every ability.

- **<u>Free Online Yoga Classes</u>**
  A playlist of free meditative yoga classes.

- **<u>Yoga with Adriene</u>**
  Free yoga videos for all levels.

Addiction Recovery Resources

- **Alcoholics Anonymous Online** Online group meetings.

- **Alcoholics Anonymous Intergroup** Online meetings directory.

- **Narcotics Anonymous Online: Never Alone Club** A Narcotics Anonymous group with daily online meetings and 24/7 support and fellowship.

- **The e-AA Group: Multi-topic Alcoholics Anonymous Forum**
  In most cases, online addiction resources are a helpful way to continue the recovery process. However, if you are suffering from withdrawal symptoms, it is important to seek professional addiction treatment. If you are concerned about how your addiction may affect your physical and mental health, call us at the number below or start a conversation in the chatbox. We offer insights and guidance based on your personal situation.

ACKNOWLEDGMENTS

Dr. Hasan Asif, thank you for the incredibly excellent work you have done with me that has contributed greatly to my recovery from both depression and anxiety. You have seen me through many ups and downs in all respects. The things I am most grateful for are you instilling in me the concept that I am more than my diagnosis. Also, your focus on a holistic approach to treating mental illness has been helpful to me, as well as the emphasis you put on psychotherapy in your work. Your strengths-based approach and our "unique" and awesome therapeutic relationship have also contributed to my success and healing process. You also instilled in me the fact that I have had, all along, the innate strength, agency, and control to contribute to my own recovery.

The following comes to mind as I write this. It is from Corey Keyes, who wrote The Mental Health Continuum: From Languishing to Flourishing in Life. He stated, "Like mental illness, mental health is more than the presence and absence of emotional states. Subjective well-being includes measures of the presence and absence of positive functioning in life…Positive functioning consists of six dimensions of psychological well-being—self-acceptance, positive relations with others, personal growth, purpose in life, environmental mastery, and autonomy."

This book was also inspired by Dr. Kay Redfield Jamison. Kay Redfield Jamison is an American clinical psychologist and writer. Her work has centered on bipolar disorder, which she has had since her early adulthood.

Author Bio

With a passion for and dedication to public service, Audrey Adade, MSW, has worked in health and human services for 12 years. Audrey is currently a Public Health Analyst/Government Project Officer with the Health Resources and Services Administration (HRSA) for the Division of Health Careers & Financial Support, Health Careers and Pipeline Brach, within the Bureau of Health Workforce.

In her last position, Audrey served as a Public Health Advisor/Government Project Officer at the Substance Abuse and Mental Health Services Administration (SAMHSA). At SAMHSA, she gained extensive experience working with federal cooperative agreements, grants, and contracts, as well as working with states, municipalities, individual school districts, universities, community organizations, and various stakeholders.

In addition to being in the federal government, Audrey's work experience includes work in journalism, non-profits, and mental health advocacy groups. She began her career as a General Assignment Reporter for a small weekly in Fairfield, Connecticut. The best experiences she had in journalism were performing the basic tasks of interviewing people from different walks of life. Journalism taught her that everyone has a story. She then went on to work as a health outreach coordinator and patient advocate for the Sickle Cell Disease Association of America (SCDAA) Southern Connecticut, Inc. At SCDAA Southern, Connecticut, Inc., she led an initiative that created after-school educational workshops that targeted high school students. In collaboration with area schools, she provided sickle cell disease education and sickle cell screening. The purpose was the early identification of sickle cell traits in young people. She also served as a board member with the Fairfield, Connecticut chapter of the National Alliance on Mental Illness (NAMI). NAMI is the nation's largest grassroots health organization dedicated to improving the lives of people with serious mental illnesses and their families.

Her participation in NAMI changed her life. It is there she identified her strong desire to make an impact on mental health parity through public policy that positively impacts those affected by mental disabilities. Audrey also exhibited this passion through her work in behavioral health disparities at SAMHSA. She co-created a toolkit and co-led an effort to require all SAMHSA grantees to submit Disparity Impact Statements, as directed by the HHS Action Plan to Reduce Racial and Ethnic Health Disparities. This toolkit is used across agency staff, including government project officers and other program staff, grants management, grants review, and leadership.

Audrey completed her undergraduate education at Fairfield University, with a B.A. in English, concentrating in Journalism. Her graduate education was at the Columbia University School of Social Work, with an M.S. in Social Work and a concentration in Public Policy. Her area of focus was health, mental health, and disabilities.

Lastly, Audrey is the founder and CEO of ASCWA Consulting, LLC ®, an organization that provides writing and art consultation services to youth, young adults, and professionals alike. In line with her passion for service, the organization's mission is to support educational and professional growth.

Audrey can be found online at ASCWA Consulting ® on all social media platforms.

THANK YOU TO THE READER

To the reader, envision the future of your communities, and encourage the mentally ill to step into their full potential so they can see how beautiful their lives can be when they feel open and free, and are living true to themselves. What is your purpose? I found mine.

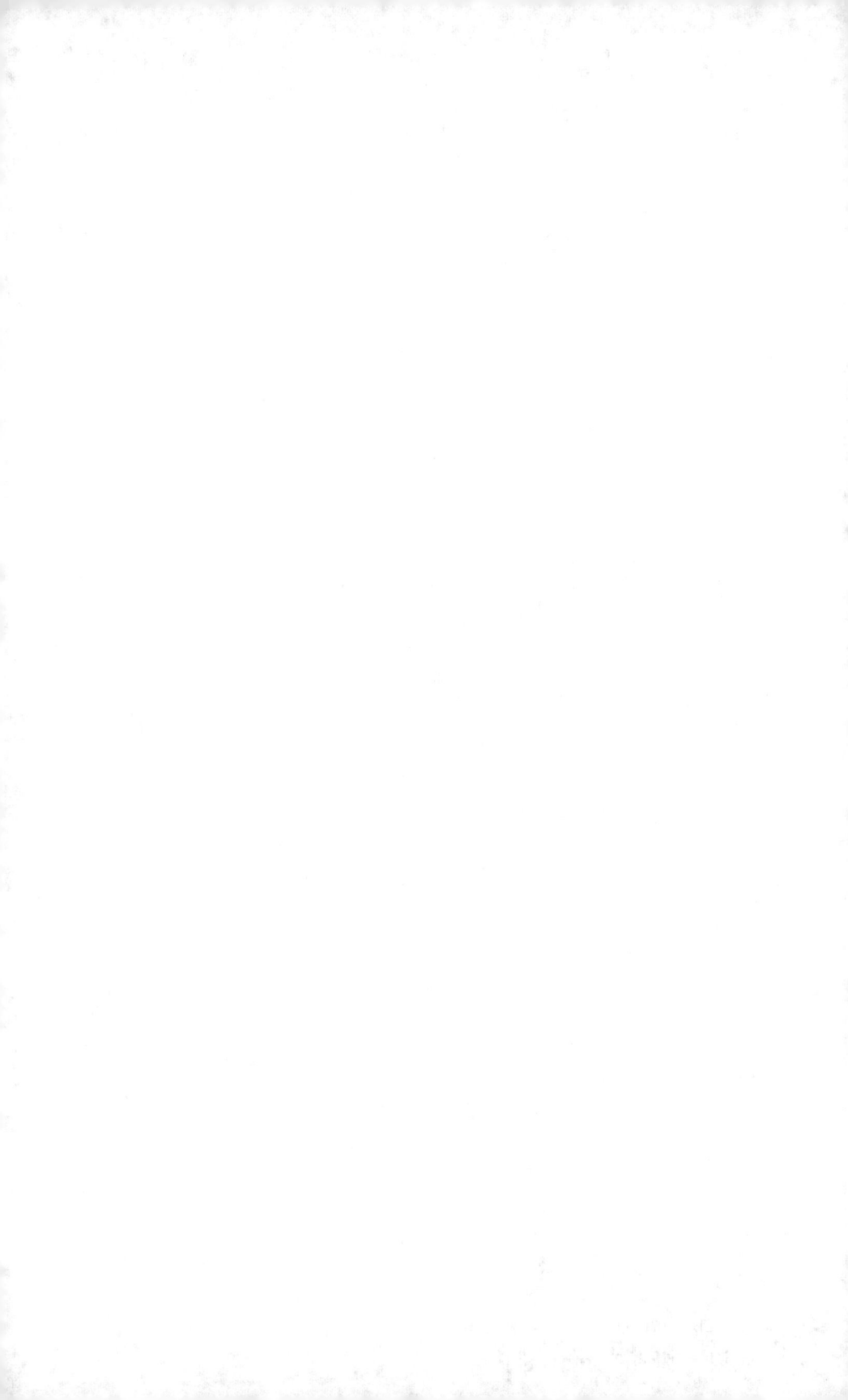

www.ingramcontent.com/pod-product-compliance
Lightning Source LLC
Chambersburg PA
CBHW060411290526
45791CB00002B/696